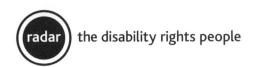 the disability rights people

National Key Scheme Guide 2011

Accessible Toilets for Disabled People

Compiled by John Stanford
11th Edition © Radar Promotions Ltd

National Key Scheme Guide 2011
Accessible Toilets for Disabled People

ISBN 978-0-9561995-9-1
13th edition © Radar Promotions Ltd 2011

Published by Radar Promotions Ltd for Radar (The Royal Association for Disability Rights) Registered Charity No. 273150

Design: © Anderson Fraser Partnership, London
Printed & bound by: Cambrian Printers Ltd, Aberystwyth

Radar
12 City Forum
250 City Road
London EC1V 8AF

Tel: 020 7250 3222
Fax: 020 7250 0212
Textphone: 020 7250 4119
www.radar.org.uk

Mixed Sources
Product group from well-managed forests and other controlled sources
www.fsc.org Cert no. TT-COC-2200
© 1996 Forest Stewardship Council
FSC

Local authorities and other providers of public toilets supply most of the information and this is supported by information and feedback from individuals, local access guides and other sources. I would like to thank everyone involved for their assistance and our advertisers for their support.

All information is provided in good faith but Radar cannot be held responsible for any omissions or inaccuracies. We have tried to get information from all organisations who may provide NKS toilets but this has not always been forthcoming. We would therefore, be pleased to hear of any additions or amendments that we can use to update our records and include in future editions.

John Stanford, Editor

CONTENTS

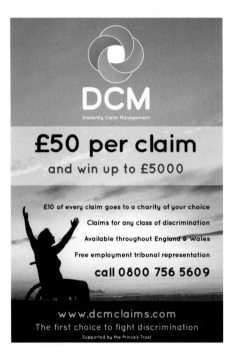
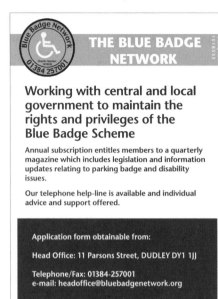
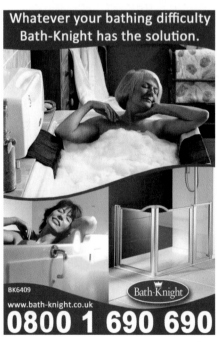
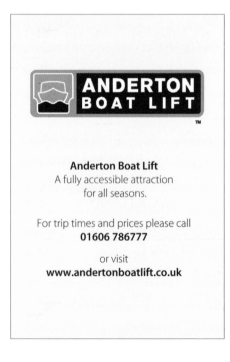

PREFACE

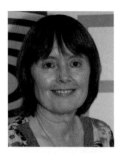

Radar is a leading UK pan-disability organisation. We believe that everyone who experiences ill-health, injury or disability should have the same freedom and independence as other citizens. We need changes in our society to achieve that – from better independent living and social care support – to routes out of poverty.

Radar campaigns on all these issues – working in Parliament, with policy makers and with many other organisations to achieve these changes. We produce a wide range of resources, guides and reports, written by and for disabled people, to share advice, encourage leadership development and promote good policy and practice for policy-makers, the public sector and business.

One important part of freedom is having the confidence to go out, knowing that public toilets will be available that are accessible and meet your needs. This guide will provide you with everything you need to know about the National Key Scheme toilets around the country.

Liz Sayce OBE
Chief Executive
Radar

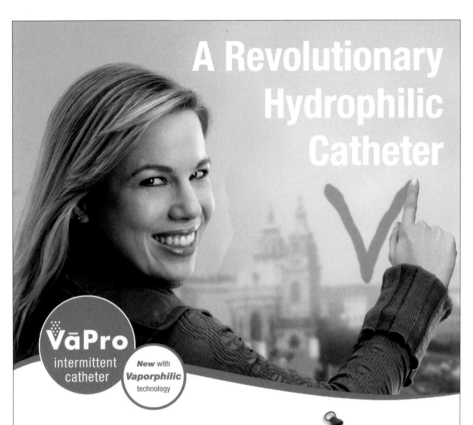

A Revolutionary Hydrophilic Catheter

VāPro intermittent catheter — *New* with *Vaporphilic* technology

A world first from Hollister, the **VaPro** intermittent catheter uses sterile water vapour to activate the catheter coating, making the catheter ready to use right out of the packaging, with no need to add water.

The catheter is designed to be:
- **Ready to use**
- **Spill-free**
- **Hygienic**

There's more to Hollister
Continence Care than ever before

More choices. More solutions. More from the heart of Hollister.

To discover more about the benefits the **VaPro intermittent catheter** can offer you, why not request some FREE samples for your own evaluation.

Visit: www.cathetersample.co.uk
Freephone: 0800 521377
e-mail: samples.uk@hollister.com

Ensure that VaPro is always used in accordance with the directions for use. Hollister and logo, Vapro and "Attention to Detail. Attention to Life." are trademarks of Hollister Incorporated. ©2011 Hollister Incorporated. CONT0038.

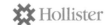 Hollister

Attention to Detail. Attention to Life.

HOW TO USE THIS GUIDE

The 2011 edition of this guide includes approaching 9,000 NKS toilets across the country. While some councils have closed a number of their public conveniences for disabled people or transferred them to other providers, increased provision by other organisations means that the number of NKS toilets increases by about one every working day.

Toilets listed are those we have been told are fitted with the NKS lock. It is not a list of all public toilets designed for disabled people.

Order of entries
Toilets locations are listed by:
- Region of the country
- District or borough council area (in alphabetical order)
- Locality (towns and villages)

Finding an NKS toilet
Within local authority districts or borough council areas, localities (towns and villages) are listed first, in alphabetical order. Locations of toilets provided by the relevant Council are then shown (alphabetically), followed by locations of toilets provided by other organisations.

An index of localities is provided at the back of this book. It includes all towns and villages but not all the localities within large towns and cities included in the main listings. For example Edinburgh is listed in the index but not the 11 individual areas of the city.

Information in entries

Opening times
Many toilets listed are available to NKS keyholders at all times. You can assume that most of the non-council toilets are not available on a 24-hour basis. Where possible, we indicate opening times, for example:
* (08.00-20.00), (Summer) or (Park hrs)

Some entries are for new toilets, planned but not yet open or those due to close at some point in the future. These are indicated by, for example:
* [Summer 11], [Proposed], or [to be replaced]

Gender
The majority of toilets are unisex. Those which are not, are indicated by:
* (M), (F), (M+F)

Number of NKS toilets available
At some locations, there is more than one NKS toilet.
* This is indicated by a number in brackets after the location.

Rural areas
In some rural areas specific details of locations are not available. It should be assumed that in those localities the location of the toilet will be obvious.
* These are indicated by: [No specific information available]

Changing Places toilets
* **CP** indicates NKS key required
* **CP** indicates NKS key not required

Toilet providers
Most toilets fitted with the NKS lock are run by the district or borough council in whose area they are located. Other providers include public authorities such as parish and county councils, commercial bodies including shopping centres, public houses, rail companies and a wide variety of other public and voluntary organisations.

An indication of the ownership of the non-district council toilets is given at the end of the entry, for example:
- *(National Trust)*, *(ScotRail)* or *(Nandos)*
- In other instances *(Private)* has been used

Some of the provider names have been abbreviated, for example:
J D Wetherspoon pubs (JDW); National Park (NP); Greater Manchester Passenger Transport Executive (GMPTE); Mitchells *&* Butlers (M&B) and Transport for London (TfL).

Although some of these toilets can be considered ordinary public conveniences, in most cases they are provided for the customers/users of the premises and are not available, as a right, to the public. They will also only usually be available when the premises are open.

REGION

District

Locality	**CP** Location (10:00-16:00) (M+F)
	Location (3) *(Private)*
	'Pub or Restaurant', Location *(JDW)*
Locality	[No specific information available]
Locality	**CP** Location (1) *(Private)*
	Shopping Centre, Location *(Shopping Centre)*
	Toilet Provider (8) *(Private)*

Examples
Above: an illustration of the abbreviations, terms and colour coding used in the listing and explained on these pages. See pages 14 and 15 for details of the areas included in each region.

Regions and the areas they include

● **Greater London**
The London boroughs of Greater London and a Central London area, (roughly that within the Congestion Charge area) including the City of London and parts of Camden, Islington, Lambeth, Southwark and Westminster.

● **South East England**
East Sussex, Kent, Surrey and West Sussex.

● **Southern England**
Berkshire, Buckinghamshire, Hampshire, the Isle of Wight and Oxfordshire.

● **West Country**
Gloucestershire, Somerset, Wiltshire, Dorset and the area around Bristol.

● **Devon & Cornwall**

● **Eastern England**
Bedfordshire, Cambridgeshire, Essex, Hertfordshire, Norfolk and Suffolk.

● **East Midlands**
Derbyshire, Leicestershire, Lincolnshire, Northamptonshire and Nottinghamshire and the southern part of the area that used to form Humberside.

● **West Midlands**
Herefordshire, Shropshire, Staffordshire, Warwickshire, West Midlands and Worcestershire.

● **North West England**
Cheshire, Cumbria, Greater Manchester, Lancashire and Merseyside.

● **Yorkshire**
North, South and West Yorkshire and the East Riding of Yorkshire and Kingston-upon-Hull districts.

● **North East England**
Durham, Northumberland and Tyne & Wear and the Tees Valley.

● **South East Scotland**
Edinburgh, Falkirk, the Lothians and the Scottish Borders.

● **South West Scotland**
Ayrshire, Dumfries & Galloway, Dunbartonshire, Lanarkshire, Renfrewshire and Glasgow.

● **East Scotland**
Aberdeenshire, Angus, Clackmannan, Fife, Perth & Kinross and Stirling.

● **Highlands & Islands of Scotland**
Argyle & Bute, Highlands, Moray, Orkney, Shetland and the Western Isles.

● **North Wales**
Anglesey, Conwy, Denbighshire, Flintshire and Gwynedd.

● **Mid & West Wales**
Carmarthenshire, Ceredigion, Pembrokeshire and Powys.

● **South Wales**
The area that formed the counties of Glamorgan and Gwent including Cardiff and Swansea.

● **Northern Ireland**

● **Channel Islands**

● **Isle of Man**

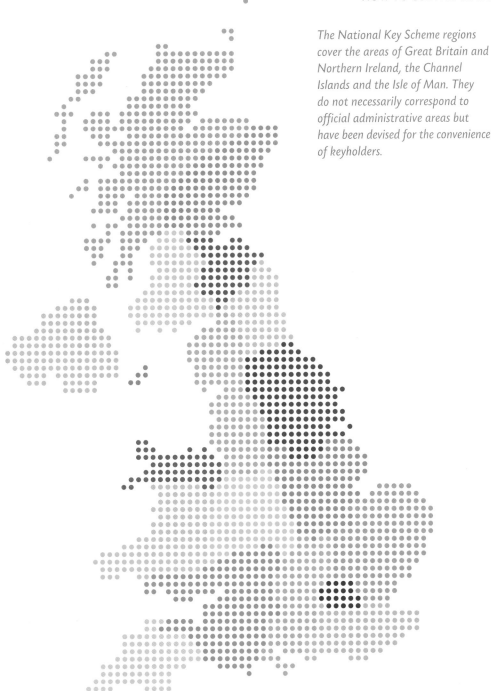

The National Key Scheme regions cover the areas of Great Britain and Northern Ireland, the Channel Islands and the Isle of Man. They do not necessarily correspond to official administrative areas but have been devised for the convenience of keyholders.

Books which open doors to independent living

To help people with lived experience of disability or health conditions lead as independent a life as possible. Radar has published two valuable guides.

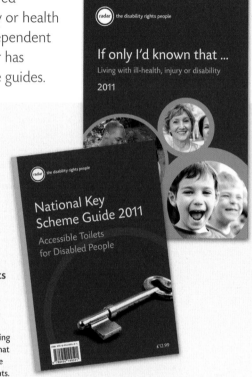

If Only I'd Known That A Year Ago 2011

A guide for everyone living with experience of disability or health conditions, their family and friends. A self-help guide signposting to valuable support and specialist information on employment, education, welfare benefits and your rights.

National Key Scheme Guide (NKS) 2011: accessible toilets for disabled people

A guide to almost 9,000 accessible disabled toilets around the UK fitted with the National Key Scheme lock. An important part of freedom is having the confidence to go out, knowing that public toilets will be available that are accessible and meet your requirements.

Buy now from Radar's online shop: www.radar-shop.org.uk

Telephone: 020 7250 3222
Textphone: 020 7250 4119
Email: radar@radar.org.uk
www.radar.org.uk

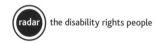

GREATER LONDON

Central London

London E1	Spitalfields Market (Trading hrs) *(Private)* 'Nandos', Middlesex Street *(Nandos)* 'Nandos', 114 Commercial Street *(Nandos)* 'Shooting Star', Middlesex Street *(Fullers)* 'Slug & Lettuce', Stoney Lane *(Private)*
London EC1	City Road/Central Street *(Islington)* Clerkenwell Road/Leather Lane *(Camden)* Long Lane, Aldersgate St *(City of London)* West Smithfield *(City of London)* Finsbury Leisure Centre (Centre hrs) *(Islington)* 'Bar 38', St Johns Street *(Private)* 'Butchers Hook & Cleaver', Smithfield *(Fullers)* 'Lord Raglan', St Martin-Le-Grand *(Private)* 'Printworks', Farringdon Road *(JDW)* 'Sir John Oldcastle', Farringdon Road *(JDW)* 'Three Compasses', Cowcross Street *(Private)*
London EC2	Liverpool St Station, Platform 10 *(Network Rail)* Bishopsgate Institute (Centre hrs) *(Private)* 'All Bar One', Finsbury Pavement *(M&B)* 'Caffe Nero', London Wall *(Private)* 'Green Man', Poultry *(JDW)* 'Hamilton Hall', Liverpool St. Station *(JDW)* 'Rack & Tenter', Moorfields *(Private)* 'The Wren', Liverpool St Station *(Private)* Guildhall School of Music (Concert hrs) *(Private)*
London EC3	Monument *(City of London)* Tower Place *(City of London)* Fenchurch Street Station, Lower Level *(Network Rail)* 'All Bar One', Houndsditch *(M&B)* 'Bar 38', St Clare House, Minories *(Private)* 'Caffe Nero', London St, Fenchurch St *(Private)* 'Crosse Keys', Gracechurch Street *(JDW)* 'Fine Line' Monument Street *(Fullers)* 'Liberty Bounds', Trinity Square *(JDW)* 'Slug & Lettuce', St Mary Axe *(Private)*

London EC4	New Change, St Paul's Churchyard *(City of London)*
	Paternoster Square **(Daytime)** *(City of London)*
	Blackfriars Station, Concourse *(Capital Connect)*
	Cannon Street Station, Lower Concourse *(Network Rail)*
	'Alibi', Shoe Lane *(Private)*
	'All Bar One', Ludgate Hill *(M&B)*
	'The Banker', Cousin Lane *(Fullers)*
	'Costa', New Bridge Street *(Costa)*
	'Fine Line', Bow Churchyard *(Fullers)*
	'Hog's Head', Fetter Lane *(Private)*
	'Leon', Ludgate Circus *(Private)*
	'The Paternoster', Paternoster Square *(Private)*
London N1	Kings Cross Station, Platform 8 *(Network Rail)*
	'Nandos', 16 York Way *(Nandos)*
London NW1	Marylebone Rd, opp. Planetarium *(Westminster)*
	Regents Park (M+F) (4) *(Royal Parks)*
	Marylebone Station, Concourse *(Chiltern Railways)*
	'Globe', Marylebone Road *(Private)*
	'Metropolitan Bar', Station Approach *(JDW)*
London SE1	Gabriels Wharf *(Private)*
	London Bridge Station, Forecourt *(Network Rail)*
	London Bridge Station, Platforms 5/6 *(Network Rail)*
	Waterloo East Station, Platform B/C *(SE Rlwy)*
	Waterloo Station, Concourse & Forecourt *(Network Rail)*
	'All Bar One', London Bridge Street *(M&B)*
	'Founders Arms', Hopton Street *(Youngs)*
	'Market Porter', Stoney Street *(Private)*

	'Nandos', Clink Street *(Nandos)*
CP	City Hall, Queens Walk (Office hrs)
CP	Tate Modern (Gallery hrs)

London SW1	Bressenden Place/Victoria Street *(Westminster)*
	Broad Sanctuary (7.30-23.00) *(Westminster)*
	Tachbrook Street (7.30-23.00) *(Westminster)*
	Victoria Place, Eccleston Bridge *(Private)*
	Victoria Coach Station, Help Point (2) *(TfL)*
	Victoria Station (2) *(Network Rail)*
	Cabinet War Rooms *(Private)*
	Caffe Nero, Haymarket *(Caffe Nero)*
	'Ha! Ha! Bar', Cardinal Walk *(Private)*
	'Lord Moon of The Mall', Whitehall *(JDW)*
	'Nandos', Cardinal Walk *(Nandos)*
	'Nandos', 107 Wilton Road *(Nandos)*
	'Shakespeare', Buckingham Palace Rd *(Private)*
	'Travellers Tavern', Elizabeth Street *(Private)*
	'Willow Walk', Wilton Road *(JDW)*

| **London SW7** | Kensington Rd, nr. Palace Gate (10.00-18.00) *(Westminster)* |
| | Mount Gate (M+F) *(Royal Parks)* |

London W1	Balderton St, off Oxford Street *(Westminster)*
	Marble Arch Subway (10.00-23.00) *(Westminster)*
	Paddington St Gardens (Daytime) *(Westminster)*
	Piccadilly Circus Station *(Westminster)* [Steps on approach]
	Regent Street/Princes Street *(Westminster)*
	Plaza Centre, 1st Floor, Oxford Street *(Private)*
	Selfridges Store, Oxford Street *(Selfridges)*

'Duke of Wellington', Wardour St *(Private)*
'Nandos', 113 Baker Street *(Nandos)*
'Nandos', Berners Street *(Nandos)*
'Nandos', Frith Street *(Nandos)*
'Nandos', Glasshouse Street *(Nandos)*
'Nandos', Googe Street *(Nandos)*
'O'Neills', Gt Marlborough Street *(M&B)*
'O'Neills', Wardour Street *(M&B)*

London W2
Paddington Station, Platform 1 *(Network Rail)*
Hyde Park, Bandstand *(Royal Parks)*
Hyde Park, Reservoir *(Royal Parks)*
'Garfunkels', Praed Street *(Private)*
'McDonalds', Edgware Road *(McDonalds)*
'Shish', Bishops Bridge Rd *(Private)*
'Tyburn', Edgware Road *(JDW)*
Grosvenor Victoria Casino, Edgware Rd *(Private)*

London WC1
High Holborn, opp Proctor Street *(Camden)*
Russell Square, opp Bernard Street *(Camden)*
'All Bar One', New Oxford Street *(M&B)*
'Marquis Cornwallis', Russell Square *(Private)*
'Nandos', Brunswick Centre *(Nandos)*
'Nandos', Southampton Place *(Nandos)*
'Pendrells Oak', High Holborn *(JDW)*
CP Great Ormond Street Hospital *(NHS Trust)*

London WC2
CP Embankment, by Underground (7.30-23.00) *(Westminster)*
Jubilee Hall, Covent Garden (7.30-23.00) *(Westminster)*

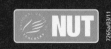

Shaftesbury Avenue, off Piccadilly Circus *(Westminster)*
Strand/Arundel Street *(Westminster)*
Charing Cross Station *(Network Rail)*
'All Bar One', Cambridge Circus *(M&B)*
'All Bar One', Kingsway *(M&B)*
'Brewmaster', Cranbourne St. *(Private)*
'Chiquito', Leicester Square *(Private)*
'Columbia Bar', Aldwych *(Private)*
'Ha! Ha! Bar', Villiers Street *(Private)*
'Knights Templar', Chancery Lane *(JDW)*
'Montagu Pyke', Charing Cross Road *(JDW)*
'Moon Under Water', Leicester Square *(JDW)*
'Nandos', Chandos Place *(Nandos)*
'Shakespeare's Head', Kingsway *(JDW)*
'Walkabout', Henrietta Street *(Private)*
'Walkabout', Temple Place *(Private)*
'Yates's Bar', Leicester Square *(Yates)*
Odeon, Leicester Square *(Odeon)*
Odeon West End, Leicester Sq *(Odeon)*
Peacock Theatre, Portugal St *(Private)*

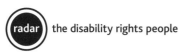

Barking & Dagenham

Barking	Barking Park, Tennis Courts (8.00-17.00)
	Clockhouse Avenue, Town Centre
	Faircross
	Fanshaw Avenue (Mon-Sat, daytime)
	Rippleside Cemetery (Mon-Sat, daytime)
	Thames View (8.00-17.00)
	Vicarage Field Shopping Centre *(Private)*
	Barking Station, Overbridge *(C2C)*
	'Barking Dog', Station Parade *(JDW)*
	'Nandos', Long Bridge Road *(Nandos)*
Chadwell Heath	Chadwell Heath Cemetery (Mon-Sat, daytime)
	St Chads Park (8.00-17.00)
	'Coopers Arms', High Road *(Private)*
Dagenham	Central Park, Pavilion (8.00-17.00)
	Eastbrookend Cemetery (Mon-Sat, daytime)
	Heathway/Hedgemans Road
	Lodge Avenue, by Mayesbrook Park
	Stamford Road (8.00-17.00)
	Dagenham Dock Station, Platform 2 *(C2C)*

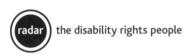

'Lord Denman', Heathway *(JDW)*
Dagenham & Redbridge FC *(Private)*

Barnet

Childs Hill	Childs Hill Park, Nant Road (Park hrs)
Colindale	'Moon Under Water', Varley Parade *(JDW)*
East Barnet	Oak Hill Park, Parkside (Park hrs) Victoria Recreation Ground, Glyn Road (Park hrs)
Edgware	Edgwarebury Park, Edgwarebury Lane (Park hrs) 'Nandos', Station Road *(Nandos)*
Finchley	Victoria Park, Ballards Lane (Park hrs) Hollywood Bowl, Gt Northern Leisure Park *(AMF)*
Friern Barnet	Friary Park, Friern Barnet Road (Park hrs)
Golders Green	Golders Hill, by Café *(City of London)* Golders Green Bus Station *(TfL)*
Hendon	Hendon Park, Queens Road (Park hrs) Sunny Hill Park (Park hrs)
High Barnet	Old Court House Recreation Ground (Café hrs)

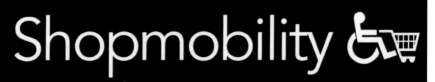

Mill Hill	Mill Hill Park, Daws Lane (Park hrs)
New Barnet	'Railway Bell', East Barnet Road *(JDW)*
North Finchley	Sainsbury's Store, 836-852 High Road *(Sainsbury)*
	'Nandos', Great North Leisure Park *(Nandos)*
	'The Tally Ho', 749 High Road *(JDW)*
Whetstone	Swan Lane Open Space, café (Café hrs)

Bexley

Abbey Wood	Lesnes Abbey (Park hrs)
	Abbey Wood Station, Booking Hall *(SE Rlwy)*
	Abbey Wood Caravan Club Site *(Caravan Club)*
Albany Park	Albany Park Station, Booking Hall *(SE Rlwy)*
Belvedere	Belvedere Recreation Ground, Heron Hill (Park hrs)
	Tower Road Campus (3) *(Bexley College)*
Bexley	Bexley Station, Platform 2 *(SE Rlwy)*
Bexleyheath	Danson Park (Park hrs)
	Danson Park Mansion (Summer, Park hrs)
	Friswell Place
	Townley Road
	The Mall Bexleyheath (2) *(Private)*
	'Furze Wren', Market Place *(JDW)*
	'The Wrong'Un', The Broadway *(JDW)*
	Gala Bingo, Broadway *(Gala)*
Blackfen	Blackfen Library (Library hrs)
Crayford	Waterside, Crayford Way
	Crayford Station, Platform 1 *(SE Rlwy)*
	'Nandos', Tower Retail Park *(Nandos)*
Erith	Town Centre
Sidcup	St John's Road
	Sidcup Station, Platform 1 *(SE Rlwy)*
	'Jolly Fenman', Blackfen Road *(Private)*
	'Tailors Chalk', Sidcup High Street *(JDW)*
	'Woodman', Blackfen Road *(Private)*
Welling	Hillview Cemetery (Cemetery hrs)
	Welling Library, Bellegrove Road (Library hrs)
	Welling Station, Platform 1 *(SE Rlwy)*
	'New Cross Turnpike', Bellegrove Rd *(JDW)*

Brent

Alperton	Douglas Avenue/Ealing Road
Brent Cross	Brent Cross Shopping Centre *(Private)* 'Nandos', Brent Cross Shopping Centre *(Nandos)*
Colindale	Oriental City Shopping Centre *(Private)*
Dollis Hill	Gladstone Park (Park hrs)
Harlesden	Harlesden Library, Craven Park Rd (Library hrs) Roundwood Park (Park hrs) Tavistock Road Car Park (8.00-17.00) Willesden Junct Station, Platform 1 *(London Overground)* 'Misty Moon', Manor Park Road *(Private)*
Kensal Rise	Chamberlayne Road/Station Terrace
Kilburn	Victoria Road/Kilburn High Street 'Caffe Nero', Kilburn High Road *(Private)* 'Nandos', Kilburn High Street *(Nandos)* Mecca Bingo, Kilburn High Rd *(Private)* Tricycle Theatre & Cinema, Kilburn High Rd *(Private)*
Kingsbury	Kingsbury Road, Car Park

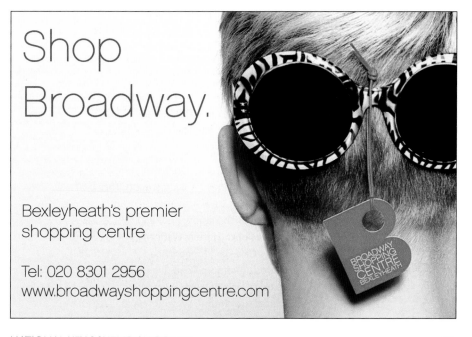

	'JJ Moons', 553 Kingsbury Road *(JDW)*
	'Nandos', Kingsbury Road *(Nandos)*
Queens Park	Car Park by Station
	Queens Park Café (Park hrs)
	Queens Park, by Playground (Park hrs)
Sudbury	Barham Park, Car Park
Wembley	Mahatma Ghandi House, Wembley Hill Road (Office hrs)
	Oakington Manor Drive/Harrow Rd (9.00-19.00)
	St Johns Road Car Park
	St Johns Road/Elm Road
	Church of the Ascension, The Avenue *(Church)*
	Paddy Power, 389 High Road *(Private)*
	'Black Horse', Harrow Road *(Private)*
	'Fusilier', 652 Harrow Road *(Private)*
	'JJ Moons', 397 High Road *(JDW)*
	'KFC', 434 High Road *(Private)*
	'McDonalds',482 High Road *(McDonalds)*
	'Nando's', 420 High Road *(Nandos)*
	'The Preston', Preston Road *(Private)*
	Wembley Arena (8) *(Private)*
	Wembley Stadium (147) *(Private)*
Willesden	High Road, off Richmond Avenue
	Quality House, Willesden Lane (Office hrs)

Bromley

Beckenham	High Street/Kelsey Park Road
	Beckenham Junction Station, Platform 2 *(SE Rlwy)*
	Clock House Station, Concourse *(SE Rlwy)*
	'Slug & Lettuce', 150 High Street *(Private)*
Bromley	The Hill, Beckenham Lane/High Street
	Library Gardens, off High Street
	Stockwell Building 2, Civic Centre (Office hrs)
	Glades MSCP, Level 2 *(Private)*
	Bromley North Station, Booking Hall *(SE Rlwy)*
	Bromley South Station, Platform 3/4 *(SE Rlwy)*
	'Henrys Café Bar', Ringers Road *(Private)*
	'Nandos', Widmore Road *(Nandos)*
	'Partridge', High Street *(Fullers)*
	'Richmal Crompton', Westmoreland Place *(JDW)*

	'Widmore Centre' Nightingale Road *(Private)*
	Churchill Theatre, High Street *(Private)*
	Empire Cinema, 2423 High Street *(Private)*
Chislehurst	High Street, Car Park
Coney Hall	Kingsway
Crystal Palace	Crystal Palace Park
	Crystal Palace Caravan Club Site *(Caravan Club)*
Farnborough	Church Road (M/F)
Locksbottom	Pallant Way, off Crofton Road
Orpington	The Walnuts Precinct, off High Street
	Priory Gardens Recreation Ground, Perry Hall Rd
	Orpington Station, Platform 3/4 *(SE Rlwy)*
	'Harvest Moon', High Street *(JDW)*
	'Nandos', Nugent Shopping Park *(Nandos)*
	Walnuts Leisure Centre *(Private)*
Penge	High Street, by McDonalds
	'McDonalds', High Street *(McDonalds)*
	'Moon & Stars', High Street *(JDW)*
Petts Wood	Station Square
	'Daylight Inn', Station Square *(Private)*
	'Sovereign of the Seas', Queensway *(JDW)*
West Wickham	Glebe Way, by Library
	West Wickham Station, Platform 1 *(SE Rlwy)*
	'Railway Hotel', Red Lodge Road *(Private)*

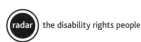

Camden (see also Central London)

Camden Town		Camden Lock Market *(Private)*
		'The Crescent', Camden High Street *(Private)*
		'Edward's'', Camden High Street *(Private)*
		'Ice Wharf', Suffolk Wharf *(JDW)*
		'Jongleurs', Camden Lock *(Private)*
Cricklewood		'Beaten Docket', Cricklewood Broadway *(JDW)*
Hampstead		Nassington Rd, Athletics Track *(City of London)*
		Vale of Health/East Heath Road *(City of London)*
Highgate		Pond Square, South Grove
		Millfield Lane, Highgate West Hill *(City of London)*
		Parliament Hill Fields *(City of London)*
Holloway	**CP**	Centre 404, Camden Road *(Private)*
Kentish Town	**CP**	Camden Society, Holmes Road (Centre hrs)
Kilburn		West End Lane/Mill Lane
Swiss Cottage		Queens Crescent/Malden Road
West Hampstead		'Walkabout', 02 Centre *(Private)*
		'Wetherspoons', O2 Centre *(JDW)*

The City Of London (See Central London)

Croydon

Coulsdon	Brighton Road, opp Chipstead Valley Rd
	Coulsdon Road, Grange Park Recreation Grnd
	Farthing Downs *(City of London)*
Croydon	Croydon Clocktower (Library & Venue hrs)
	Wellesley Road, Lunar House
	East Croydon Station Platform 3/4 *(Southern)*
	West Croydon Bus Station *(TfL)*
	'All Bar One', Park Lane *(M&B)*
	'Builders Arms', Leslie Park *(Fullers)*
	'Caffe Nero', George Street *(Private)*
	'Escapade', High Street *(Private)*
	'The George', George Street *(JDW)*
	'Goose on the Market', Surrey Street *(M&B)*
	'Milan Bar', High Street *(JDW)*
	'Nandos', 29 High Street *(Nandos)*

'Nandos', Valley Park Leisure Centre *(Nandos)*
'Porter & Sorter', Station Road East *(Marstons)*
'Ship of Fools', London Road *(JDW)*
'The Skylark', Southend *(JDW)*
'Spread Eagle', Katherine Street *(Fullers)*
'Tiger Tiger', High Street *(Private)*
'Yates's Bar', High Street *(Yates)*
Tenpin, Valley Park Leisure Centre *(Private)*

Crystal Palace
'Postal Order', Westow Street *(JDW)*
Gala Bingo, Church Road *(Gala)*

Norbury
'Moon Under Water', London Road *(JDW)*

Purley
'Foxley Hatch', Russell Hill Road *(JDW)*
Purley Bowl, Brighton Road *(Private)*

Selsdon
Monks Hill Sports Centre (Centre hrs)
Selsdon Library (Library hrs)
'Sir Julian Huxley', Addington Road *(JDW)*

South Norwood
Norwood Junction Station *(London Overground)*
'William Stanley', High Street *(JDW)*

Thornton Heath
'Flora Sandes', Brigstock Road *(JDW)*

Upper Norwood
Biggin Woods (Daytime)

Ealing

Acton
Acton Green, South Parade
'Goldsmiths Arms', East Acton Lane *(Private)*
'Red Lion & Pineapple', High Street *(JDW)*
CP Acton & W London College *(College)*

Ealing
Walpole Park *(April-September)*
Broadway Shopping Centre *(Private)*
Ealing Broadway Station *(Gt Western)*
'Fox & Goose', Hanger Lane *(Fullers)*
'The Green', The Green *(Private)*
'Nandos', Bond Street *(Nandos)*
'Rose & Crown', St Marys Road *(Fullers)*
'Sir Michael Balcon', The Mall *(JDW)*
St Marys Road Campus *(Thames Valley Univ)*

Greenford
Oldfield Lane, South Greenford

Hanwell
Brent Lodge Park (Park hrs)

Park Royal	'Nandos', Kendal Avenue *(Nandos)*
Southall	Southall Park, Southall High St
	The Broadway/Dane Road
	Ealing Hospital, Uxbridge Road *(Health Authority)*
West Ealing	Pitshanger Park
	'Drayton Court', The Avenue *(Fullers)*
	'Duke of Kent', Scotch Common *(Fullers)*

Enfield

Edmonton	Bury Lodge Gardens (Park hrs)
	Craig Park (Park hrs)
	Jubilee Park (Park hrs)
	Edmonton Green Shopping Centre *(Private)*
	'Stag & Hounds', Bury Street West *(Private)*
Enfield	Bush Hill Park (Park Hrs)
	Civic Centre (M+F) (Office hrs)
	Enfield Playing Field (Park hrs)
	Forty Hall, Forty Hill (Park hrs)
	Town Park, Cecil Road
	Palace Gardens Shopping Centre (2) *(Private)*

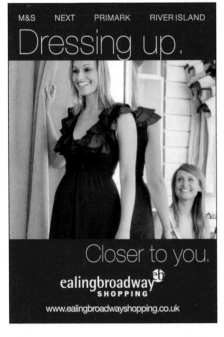
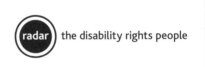

Enfield Town Station *(NX East Anglia)*
'Moon Under Water', Chase Side *(JDW)*
'Robin Hood', The Ridgeway *(Private)*
'Rose & Crown', Clay Hill *(Private)*

Enfield Highway	Albany Park, Hetford Road
	Durants Park, Hertford Road (2)
	Turkey Street/Hertford Road
New Southgate	Arnos Park (Park hrs)
North Enfield	Trent Park, Cockfosters Road
Palmers Green	Broomfield Park (2) (Park hrs)
	'Alfred Herring', Green Lanes *(JDW)*
Ponders End	Recreation Ground, High Street (2)
	'Picture Palace', Lincoln Road *(JDW)*
Southgate	Boundary Playing Fields
	Grovelands Park (Park hrs)
	Oakwood Park (Park hrs)
	Tatem Park (Park hrs)
	'New Crown', Chase Side *(JDW)*
	'White Hart', Chase Road *(Private)*
Upper Edmonton	Pymmes Park, Victoria Road
	'Gilpins Bell', Fore Street *(JDW)*

Greenwich

Abbey Wood	Bostall Gardens (Daylight)
Blackheath	Battley Park
	Blackheath Station, Platform 1 *(SE Rlwy)*
	Westcombe Park Station, Plaqtform 1 *(SE Rlwy)*
	'Royal Standard', Vanbrugh Road *(Private)*
Charlton	Charlton House (Daytime)
Eltham	Avery Hill Park, Bexley Road (Daylight)
CP	Eltham Centre (Centre hrs)
	Eltham Crematorium (Crematorium hrs)
	Eltham Park South (Daylight)
	Well Hall Pleasance (Park hrs)
	Well Hall Road
	Eltham Station, Booking Hall *(SE Rlwy)*
	New Eltham Station, Platform 1 *(SE Rlwy)*
	'Bankers Draft', High Street *(JDW)*

	Sparrows Farm, Avery Hill Campus *(Greenwich Univ.)*
Greenwich	Cutty Sark Gardens
	East Greenwich Library (Library hrs)
	Rodmere Street (7.00-19.00)
	St Alfege Recreation Centre (Centre hrs)
	Tourist Information Centre (Centre hrs)
	Greenwich Park, Blackheath Gate *(Royal Parks)*
	Greenwich Park, by Play Area *(Royal Parks)*
	Greenwich Station, Booking Hall *(SE Rlwy)*
	Maze Hill Station, Booking Hall *(SE Rlwy)*
	'Auctioneer', Greenwich High Road *(Private)*
	'Gate Clock', Creek Road *(JDW)*
	'Yacht', Crane Street *(Private)*
	Greenwich Picture House *(Private)*
Mottingham	Mottingham Station, Platform 1 *(SE Rlwy)*
North Greenwich	'Ha! Ha! Bar', Entertainment Ave., O2 *(Private)*
	'Las Iguanas', Peninsula Square *(Private)*
	'Nandos', UCI, Bugsbys Way *(Nandos)*
	'Nandos', O2, Millennium Way *(Nandos)*
	'Slug & Lettuce', Peninsula Square *(Private)*
Shooters Hill	'Fox Under the Hill', 286 Shooters Hill Road *(Private)*
	'Latin Touch Café', Oxleas Wood *(Private)*
Thamesmead	'Princess Alice', Battery Road *(Private)*
Woolwich	Beresford Square (7.00-19.00)
	The Ferry (7.00-19.00)
	Herbert Road (7.00-19.00)
	Vincent Road (7.00-19.00)
	Woolwich Arsenal Station, Platform 1 *(SE Rlwy)*
	'Earl of Chatham', Thames Street *(Private)*
	'Great Harry', Wellington Street *(JDW)*
	'McDonalds', Powis Street *(McDonalds)*
	'Nandos', Powis Street *(Nandos)*
	Gala Bingo, Powis Street *(Gala)*

Hackney

Dalston	Birkbeck Road, Ridley Road Market
	Kingsland Passage, Dalston Junction
	Kingsland Waste
	Kingsland Shopping Centre Car Park *(Private)*

	Dalston Junction Station *(London Overground)*
	Haggerston Station *(London Overground)*
	'Nandos', Kingsland High Street *(Nandos)*
Hackney	Narrow Way, Mare Street
	Wilton Way, by Town Hall
	St John at Hackney Gardens Inf. Centre *(Private)*
	'Baxters Court', Mare Street *(JDW)*
Hoxton	Hoxton Market, Stanway Street
	Hoxton Station *(London Overground)*
Stamford Hill	Stamford Hill Broadway
Stoke Newington	Clissold Park (Park hrs)
	Newington Green
	'Nandos', Church Street *(Nandos)*
	'Rochester Castle', High Street *(JDW)*

Hammersmith & Fulham

Fulham	Lillie Road/Fulham Palace Road
	Vanston Place, Fulham Broadway
	'Crabtree', Rainville Road *(Private)*
	'Durell', Fulham Road *(Private)*
	'Nandos', 20 Fulham Broadway *(Nandos)*
	'Oyster Rooms', Fulham Broadway *(JDW)*
	Craven Cottage *(Fulham FC)*
Hammersmith	Hammersmith Broadway Centre (2)
	Kings Mall Shopping Centre
	Ravenscourt Park, Café (9.30-17.30)
	Social Services Office, King Street (Office hrs)
	Talgarth Road
	'Hop Poles', King Street *(Private)*
	'Old Trout', Broadway *(Private)*
	'Plough & Harrow', King Street *(JDW)*
	'Rutland', Lower Mall *(Private)*
	'William Morris', King Street *(JDW)*
	Hammersmith Apollo *(Private)*
Shepherds Bush	Shepherds Bush Green, by Post Office
	White City Bus Station *(TfL)*
	'Central Bar', West 12 Shopping Centre *(JDW)*
	'Nandos', 284 Uxbridge Roiad *(Nandos)*
	'Nandos', Westfield Shopping Centre *(Nandos)*

'Walkabout', Shepherds Bush Green *(Private)*
Cinema, Shepherds Bush Centre *(Private)*

Haringey

Crouch End	Hatherley Gardens/Haringey Park
Finsbury Park	Finsbury Park Recreation Ground, by Café
Highgate	Highgate Wood *(City of London)* 'The Gatehouse', North Road *(JDW)*
Hornsey	'The Tollgate', Turnpike Lane *(JDW)*
Muswell Hill	Summerland Gardens Car Park
South Tottenham	Apex Corner, Seven Sisters Road St Ann's Road, Chestnut Recreation Ground
Tottenham	Tottenham Hale Station, Platform 2 *(NX East Anglia)*
Wood Green	The Mall Shopping City *(Private)* 'The Gate', Buckingham Road *(Private)* 'Wetherspoons', Spouters Corner *(JDW)*

Harrow

Edgware	Bob Lawrence Library (Library hrs) Whitchurch Lane/Buckingham Road The Mall Broadwalk, Station Road *(Private)* 'Zan Zi Bar', High Street *(Private)*
Harrow	Greenhill Way, nr. Havelock Place Harrow Leisure Centre (Centre hrs) St Anns Shopping Centre *(Private)*

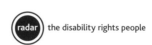

	St George's Shopping *(Private)* Harrow Bus Station *(TfL)* 'Castle', West Street *(Fullers)* 'The Junction', Gaydon Way *(Private)* 'Moon on the Hill', Station Road *(JDW)* 'Mumbai Junction', 211 Watford Road *(Private)* 'O'Neills', Station Road *(M&B)* 'Rat & Parrot', St Anns Road *(Private)* 'Yates's Bar', Station Road *(Yates)*
Harrow Weald	High Road 'Leefe Robinson VC', Uxbridge Road *(Private)*
Hatch End	'Moon & Sixpence', Uxbridge Road *(JDW)*
Kenton	Belmont Circle, Kenton Lane 'New Moon', Kenton Road *(JDW)*
North Harrow	Pinner Road
Pinner	Chapel Lane 'Caffe Nero', Love Lane *(Private)* 'Village Inn', Rayners Lane *(JDW)*
Rayners Lane	Rayners Lane, opp. Station
South Harrow	Northolt Road 'Nandos', 306 Northolt Road *(Nandos)*
Stanmore	Stanmore Recreation Ground (Park hrs) 'Crazy Horse', Church Road *(Private)* 'Man in the Moon', Buckingham Parade *(JDW)*
Sudbury Hill	'Rising Sun', Greenford Road *(Private)*
Wealdstone	Gladstone Way MSCP 'Goodwill To All', Headstone Drive *(Private)* 'Miller & Carter', Brockhurst Corner *(Private)* 'Stone Rose', High Street *(Private)*

Havering

Collier Row	Collier Row Road 'Aspen Tree', Gobions Avenue *(Greene King)* 'Bell & Gate', Collier Row Lane *(Private)* 'Colley Rowe Inn', Collier Row *(JDW)*
Corbetts Tey	'Huntsman & Hounds', Ockendon Road *(Private)*
Cranham	'Golden Crane', Avon Road *(Private)*

Elm Park	Station Parade
Gidea Park	Station Road
Harold Hill	Hilldene Avenue
Havering-atte-Bower	'Orange Tree', Orange Tree Inn *(Private)*
Hornchurch	Appleton Way 'Ardleigh & Dragon', Ardleigh Green Rd *(Private)* 'Harrow', Hornchurchg Road *(Private)* 'Hogshead', Station Lane *(Private)* 'JJ Moons', High Street *(JDW)* 'Lloyds Bar', High Street *(JDW)* 'Nandos', 306 Northolt Road *(Nandos)* 'Railway', Station Lane *(Private)*
Rainham	Cherry Tree Lane 'Albion', Rainham Road
Romford	South Street Liberty Shopping Centre *(Private)* The Mall Romford *(Private)* Debenhams Store, Market Pl *(Debenhams)* Romford Station, Platform 4 *(NX East Anglia)* 'Custom House', South Street *(Private)* 'Edwards', South Street *(Private)* 'Moon & Stars', South Street *(JDW)* 'Nandos', The Brewery *(Nandos)* 'Squire', North Street *(Private)* 'Worlds Inn', South Street *(JDW)* 'Yates's Bar', South Street *(Yates)* Rush Green Campus, Dagenham Road (6) *(College)*

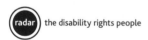

Upminster	Upminster Bridge, Upminster Road
	Upminster Station, Lower Ticket Office *(C2C)*
	'Optomist', Hacton Lane *(Private)*

Hillingdon

Cowley	Station Road
Devonshire Lodge	Car Park
Eastcote	'The Manor', Field End Road *(Private)*
Harefield	Park Lane, by Library
Hatton Cross	by Underground Station
Hayes	Barra Hall Park
	Botwell Lane
	Coldharbour Lane
	Connaught Recreation Ground
	St Anselms Road, Town Centre
	Hayes & Harlington Station *(Gt Western)*
	'Botwell Inn', Coldharbour Lane *(JDW)*
Hillingdon	'Red Lion', Royal Lane *(Fullers)*
Ickenham	Community Close
	'Titchenham Inn', Swakeleys Road *(JDW)*
Northwood	Joel Street
	Oaklands Gate
	'William Jolle', The Broadway *(JDW)*

Ruislip	High Street
	Manor Farm
	'JJ Moons', Victoria Road *(JDW)*
Ruislip Manor	Linden Avenue
Uxbridge	Fairfield Road
	The Mall Pavilions *(Private)*
	Debenhams Store, The Chimes *(Debenhams)*
	'Good Yarn', High Street *(JDW)*
	'Nandos', The Chimes *(Nandos)*
	'White House', Stockley Park *(JDW)*

Hounslow

Bedfont	Bedfont Library, Staines Road (Library hrs)
Brentford	Half Acre/Lion Way, Brentford High Street
	Brentford Station, Waiting Room *(SW Trains)*
	Syon Park, Wyevale Garden Centre *(Private)*
	Kew Bridge Steam Museum *(Private)*
Chiswick	'Hog's Head', Chiswick High Road *(Private)*
	'Nandos', 187 Chiswick High Rd *(Nandos)*
	'Packhorse & Talbot', Chiswick High Rd *(Private)*
	'Paragon', Chiswick High Road *(Private)*
	'Roebuck', Chiswick High Road *(Private)*
Cranford	'Jolly Waggoner', 618 Bath Road *(Private)*
Feltham	Feltham Library (Library hrs)
	Feltham Station, Booking Hall *(SW Trains)*
	'Moon on the Square', The Centre *(JDW)*

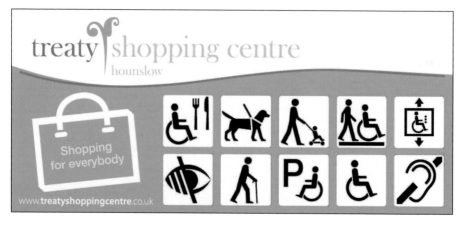

	'Nandos', Longford Shopping Centre *(Nandos)*
	Gala Bingo, Airpark Way *(Gala)*
	Hounslow Urban Farm, Fagg's Road *(Private)*
Gunnersbury	Gunnersbury Park (Park hrs)
Heston	'Rose & Crown', 220 Heston Road *(Private)*
Heston M4	Heston Services East, J2/3 M4 *(Moto)*
	Heston Services West, J2/3 M4 *(Moto)*
Hounslow	Treaty Shopping Centre (2) *(Private)*
	'Bullstrode', Lampton Road *(Private)*
	'KFC', High Street *(KFC)*
	'Moon Under Water', 84 Staines Rd *(JDW)*
	'Nandos', High Street *(Nandos)*
	'TJB's Café', Treaty Centre *(Private)*
	'Yates's Bar', Bath Road *(Yates)*
	Gala Bingo, Staines Road *(Gala)*
	Lampton Sports Centre, Lampton Avenue *(Private)*
Isleworth	'London Apprentice', Church Street *(Private)*
Osterley	'Hare & Hounds', Windmill Lane *(Private)*

Islington (see also Central London)

Archway	Archway Leisure Centre *(Centre hrs)*
Barnsbury	'Albion', Thornhill Road *(Private)*
Canonbury	'The House', Canonbury Road *(Private)*
Finsbury Park	N4 Library, Blackastock Road (Library hrs)
	Centre for Lifelong Learning, Blackstock Rd *(College)*
Highbury	Highbury Crescent, by Highbury Pool
	Highbury Fields, Tennis Courts End
	Emirates Stadium *(Arsenal FC)*
Holloway	Sobell Leisure Centre (Centre hrs)
	London Met University, Holloway Rd *(University)*
	Morrison's Store, Holloway Road *(Morrison)*
	James Selby Ltd, Holloway Road *(Private)*
	'The Coronet', Holloway Road *(JDW)*
	'McDonalds', Seven Sisters Road *(McDonalds)*
Islington	Council Offices, Upper Street (Office hrs)
	Islington Green, Essex Road
	White Conduit Street, Chapel Market (8.00-18.00)

	N1 Centre, Islington High Street *(Private)*
	'The Angel', Islington High Street *(JDW)*
	'Glass Works', N1 Centre *(JDW)*
	'Steam Passage', Upper Street *(Private)*
	'White Swan', Upper Street *(JDW)*
Stroud Green	'White Lion of Mortimer', Stroud Green Rd *(JDW)*

Kensington & Chelsea

Earls Court	'McDonalds', Earls Court Road *(McDonalds)*
Kensington	Holland Park, Ilchester Place (Park hrs)
	Kensington High Street, by Odeon
	Kensington Town Hall Car Park (Daytime)
North Kensington	Emslie Hornimans Pleasance, Bosworth Rd (Park hrs)
	Portobello Road/Lonsdale Road
Notting Hill	Kensington Memorial Park, St Marks Rd (Park hrs)
	Notting Hill Gate, opp. Cinema
	Tavistock Piazza
	Westbourne Grove/Colville Road
	'Duke of Wellington', Portobello Road *(Youngs)*
	'The Mitre', Holland Park Avenue *(Private)*
	'Nandos', Notting Hill Gate *(Nandos)*
South Kensington	'Black Widow', Gloucester Road *(Private)*
	'Nandos', 117 Gloucester Road *(Nandos)*
West Brompton	Westfield Park
West Kensington	Kensington Olympia Station, Booking Hall *(London Overgrnd)*
	'Kensington', Russell Gardens *(Private)*

Kingston-Upon-Thames

Chessington	Hook & Chessington Library, Hook Rd (Library hrs)
	'Chessington Oak', Moore Lane *(M&B)*
	'North Star', Hook Road *(Private)*
Kingston	Barnfield Youth & Community Centre (Centre hrs)
	Bittoms Car Park (Mon-Sat, 7.45-19.00)
	Eden Walk Car Park, by Shopmobility
	Guildhall 1, Foyer (Office hrs)
	Guildhall 2, Ground floor (Office hrs)
	Kingston Crematorium (Opening hrs)
	Kingsmeadow Fitness Centre (Centre hrs)
	Market Hall, Market Place
	The Rose Car Park, Kingston Hall Road
	Kingston College, Richmond Road *(College)*
	Cromwell Street Bus Station *(TfL)*
	Kingston Station, Platform 2 *(SW Trains)*
	Bentalls Centre *(Private)*
	John Lewis Store, Wood Street *(John Lewis)*
	'The Ballroom', Oceana *(Private)*
	'British Oak', Richmond Road *(Private)*
	'Departure Lounge', Oceana *(Private)*
	'Frangos', The Rotunda *(Private)*
	'Ha! Ha! Bar', Charter Quay *(Private)*
	'King's Tun', Clarence Street (2) *(JDW)*
	'Kingston Mill', High Street *(M&B)*
	'Litten Tree', Castle Street *(Private)*
	'McDonalds', Eden Street *(McDonalds)*

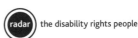 the disability rights people

Doing Money Differently

Part of our 'Doing Life Differently' series, this toolkit explores new ways of making, saving and looking after your money.

Available from Radar's online shop
www.radar-shop.org.uk

	'Oceana', Clarence Street *(Private)*
	'O'Neill's', Eden Street *(M&B)*
	'Slug & Lettuce', Charter Quay *(Private)*
	Gala Bingo, Richmond Road *(Gala)*
	Hawker Leisure Centre *(YMCA)*
New Malden	Blagdon Road Car Park
	Malden Centre, Cocks Crescent
	New Malden Library, Kingston Rd (Library hrs)
	'Bar Malden', St Georges Square *(Marstons)*
	'The Fountain', Malden Road *(Private)*
CP	Crescent Resource Centre (Cerntre hrs)
Norbiton	'Kingston Gate', London Road *(Private)*
Surbiton	Claremont Road, by Clocktower
	Victoria Recreation Ground
	Surbiton Station, Platforms *(SW Trains)*
	'Cap in Hand', Hook Rise *(JDW)*
	'Coronation Hall', St Marks Hill *(JDW)*
	'Elm Tree', Victoria Street *(Private)*
	'Rat & Parrot', St Marks Hill *(Private)*
	'Surbiton Flyer', Victoria Road *(Fullers)*
Tolworth	Alexandra Recreation Ground
	Tolworth Recreation Centre *(Private)*
	'Broadway Café Bar', The Broadway *(Marstons)*
	Charrington Bowl, Kingston Road *(AMF)*

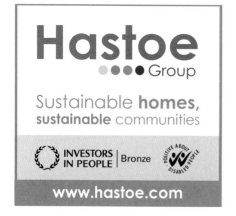

Lambeth (see also Central London)

Brixton	Popes Road
	'The Beehive', 407 Brixton Road *(JDW)*
Clapham	'Revolution', Clapham High Street *(Private)*
Herne Hill	Herne Hill Station, Platform 3 *(SE Rlwy)*
Streatham	The Rookery, Streatham Common
	'Crown & Sceptre', Streatham Hill Rd *(JDW)*
	'Holland Tringham', High Road *(JDW)*
	'Nandos', 6 The High Parade *(Nandos)*
Vauxhall	Vauxhall Bus Station *(TfL)*
West Norwood	Norwood High Street, by Library

Lewisham

Blackheath	Blackheath Grove
	'The Railway', Blackheath Village *(Private)*
Brockley	'Brockley Barge', Brockley Road *(JDW)*
Catford	Catford Broadway/Catford Grove
	Catford Bridge Station, Platform 2 *(SE Rlwy)*
	'London & Rye', Rushey Green *(JDW)*
	'Nandos', Rushey Green *(Nandos)*
Deptford	Brookmill Park (Park hrs)
	Giffin Street (7.00-19.00)
Downham	Downham Way/Old Bromley Road
Forest Hill	Forest Hill Station Forecourt
	'The Capitol', London Road *(JDW)*
Grove Park	Chinbrook Road
	Grove Park Station, Platform 2/3 *(SE Rlwy)*
Hither Green	'Station Hotel', Hither Green *(Private)*
Kidbrooke	Kidbrooke Station, Platform 1 *(SE Rlwy)*
Lee	Lee Station, Platform 1 *(SE Rlwy)*
	'The Crown', Burnt Ash Hill *(Youngs)*
	'Nando's', Lee High Road *(Nandos)*
Lee Green	Sainsbury's Store, Burnt Ash Rd *(Sainsbury)*
	'Edmund Halley', Lee Gate Centre *(JDW)*
Lewisham	Lewisham High Street, by Littlewoods

Lewisham Library (Library hrs)
Lewisham Shopping Centre *(Private)*
Lewisham Station, Platform 2/3 *(SE Rlwy)*
'Market Tavern', High Street *(Marstons)*
'Marlowes', High Street *(Private)*
'Watch House', High Street *(JDW)*

New Cross
New Cross Station, Platform A/B *(SE Rlwy)*
'Hobgoblin', New Cross Road *(Private)*

Sydenham
Home Park
Sydenham Station Approach
'Two Halfs', Sydenham Road *(Private)*

Merton

Colliers Wood
Colliers Wood Recreation Ground
Wandle Park, Home Park Road
'Nandos', Tandem Centre *(Nandos)*

Merton Park
John Innes Park, Church Path

Mitcham
Canons Recreation Ground, Madeira Road
Rowan Road Recreation Ground
Tamworth Farm Recreation Ground, London Road
'White Lion of Mortimer', London Road *(JDW)*

Morden
Joseph Hood Recreation Ground, Martin Way
King George's Playing Field, Tudor Drive
Morden Park, London Road

Motspur Park
Sir Joseph Hood Playing Fields (Park hrs)

Raynes Park
Cottenham Park Recreation Ground
'Edward Rayne', Coombe Lane *(JDW)*

Roehampton
Commons Extension, Robin Hood Lane

West Wimbledon
Holland Gardens

Wimbledon
The Broadway/Queens Road (Daytime)
Cannizaro Park, West Side (Park hrs)
Dundonald Recreation Ground
Haydons Road Recreation Ground
South Park Gardens, Dudley Road
Wimbledon Park, Home Park Road (Park hrs)
Centre Court Shopping Centre *(Private)*
Debenhams Store, Centre Court *(Debenhams)*
Wimbledon Station, Platforms 1&8 *(SW Trains)*

'Nandos', Russell Road *(Nandos)*
'O'Neill's', The Broadway *(M&B)*
'Wibbas Down Inn', Gladstone Road *(JDW)*

Newham

Beckton	Beckton Park North (Park hrs)
	St John's Road Car Park
	Asda Superstore *(Asda)*
	'Nandos', Gallions Reach Shopping Park *(Nandos)*
Canning Town	Rathbone Market, Barking Road
	Docklands Campus *(Univ of E. London)*
East Ham	Central Park, Cafe (Park hrs)
	Clements Road/High Street North
	Plashet Park (Park hrs)
	Town Hall (Office hrs)
CP	East Ham Leisure Centre, Barking Road
	East Ham Campus, High St South *(Newham College)*
	'Millers Well', 419 Barking Road *(JDW)*
	Gala Bingo, Barking Road *(Gala)*
Forest Gate	Romford Road/Woodgrange Road
	Shaftesbury Road Car Park
	'Hudson Bay', Upton Lane *(JDW)*
Manor Park	Romford Road/Herbert Road
	City of London Cemetery (2) *(City of London)*
Plaistow	Greengate Street/Barking Road
	Hamara Ghar Square
	Queens Market
CP	Community Centre, Balaam Street
	Boleyn Ground, Upton Park *(West Ham Utd)*
Stratford	Stratford Campus, Welfare Road *(Newham College)*
	Stratford Shopping Centre *(Private)*
	Stratford Station *(TfL)*
	'Golden Grove', The Grove *(JDW)*
	'Goose on the Broadway', Broadway *(M&B)*
	'Nandos', 1a Romford Road *(Nandos)*
	'Swan', The Broadway *(Private)*
	Gala Bingo, High Street *(Gala)*
West Ham	West Ham Park *(City of London)*

Redbridge

Barkingside	Cranbrook Rd, by Park
	'New Fairlop Oak', Fencepiece Road *(JDW)*
	Gala Bingo, Fairlop Road *(Gala)*
Chadwell Heath	Wangey Road (7.30-21.00)
	'Eva Hart', High Street *(JDW)*
Clayhall	Clayhall Park, Longwod Gdns
Gants Hill	Clarence Avenue (7.30-21.00)
Goodmayes	High Road/Barley Lane (Mon-Sat, 7.30-18.30)
Hainault	Hainault Recreation Ground (Park hrs)
	Manford Way
Ilford	Cranbrook Road, nr. The Drive (Mon-Sat, 7.30-18.30)
	Chapel Road/Roden Street
	Horns Road, op.B&Q (Mon-Sat, 7.30-18.30)
	Ilford Central Library (Library hrs)
	Ilford High Road, Griggs Approach
	Ley Street, MSCP
	The Mall Ilford (3) *(Private)*

Clements Road MSCP *(Private)*
Ilford Station, Overbridge *(NX East Anglia)*
'Great Spoon of Ilford', Cranbrook Rd *(JDW)*
'Nandos', Clements Road *(Nandos)*

Seven Kings	Aldborough Rd South, opp. Chepstow Cres (Mon-Sat) High Road, nr Station Car Park (Mon-Sat, 7.30-18.30) South Park Road, off Green Lane (7.30-18.30)
South Woodford	Eastwood Close
Wanstead	Christchurch Green, off High St (M+F) (7.30-21.00) Wanstead Park *(City of London)* 'Cuckfield', High Street *(Private)* 'The George', High Street *(JDW)*
Woodford Green	Hillside Avenue Johnston Road

Richmond-Upon-Thames

Barnes	'Red Lion', Castelnau *(Fullers)*
Hampton	Bushy Park, by Playground *(Royal Parks)* Hampton Court Palace, Tiltyard Restaurant *(Private)*
Richmond	Buccleuch Gardens, off Petersham Road Old Town Hall, Whitaker Avenue Princes Street, behind Waitrose Victoria Place Richmond Station, Lower Level *(SW Trains)* Sainsburys Store, Manor Road *(Sainsbury)* 'Bull', 1 Kew Road *(Private)* 'Edwards', Kew Road *(M&B)* 'The Lot', Duke Street *(Private)* 'New Inn', Petersham Road *(Private)* 'Old Ship', King Street *(Youngs)* 'O'Neills', The Quadrant *(M&B)* 'Orange Tree', Kew Road *(Youngs)*
Teddington	'The Lion', Wick Road *(Private)*
Twickenham	Twickenham Station, Platform 3 *(SW Trains)* 'George', King Street *(Private)* 'Hook Line & Sinker', York Street *(Fullers)* 'William Webb Ellis', London Road *(JDW)* 'St Margaret', St Margarets Road *(Private)*

| Whitton | Whitton Library Car Park |
| | Whitton Sports & Fitness Centre (Centre hrs) |

Southwark (see also Central London)

Bermondsey	'All Bar One', Butlers Wharf *(M&B)*
	'Pommelers Rest', Tower Bridge Rd *(JDW)*
CP	Southwark College, Keetons Road *(College)*
Camberwell	'Fox on the Hill', Denmark Hill *(JDW)*
	Gala Bingo, Camberwell Road *(Gala)*
Dulwich	Dulwich Park, Pavilion Café (Park hrs)
East Dulwich	Sainsbury's Store, Dog Kennel Hill *(Sainsbury)*
Elephant & Castle	'Rockingham Arms', Metro Central Heights *(JDW)*
Peckham	'Kentish Drovers', Peckham High St *(JDW)*
Rotherhithe	Southwark Park Café (Park hrs)
	Surrey Quays Retail Park (2) *(Private)*
	'Quebec Curve', Redriff Road *(Marstons)*
	'Surrey Docks', Lower Road *(JDW)*
	Gala Bingo, Surrey Quays *(Gala)*

Sutton

Carshalton	Grove Park, by Café (Daytime)
	Oaks Park (Daytime)
Cheam	Cheam Park, Cheam Park Way (Daytime)
	Nonsuch Park, by Mansion Café *(Epsom & Ewell Council)*
North Cheam	'Nonsuch Inn', 552 London Road *(JDW)*
	'Woodstock', Stonecot Hill *(Private)*
Rosehill	Mecca Bingo, Bishopsford Road *(Mecca)*
Sutton	St Nicholas Centre (2) *(Private)*
	Morrisons Store, High Street *(Morrisons)*
	'Caffe Nero', Carshalton Road *(Private)*
	'Cock & Bull', High Street *(Fullers)*
	'The Grapes', High Street *(JDW)*
	'Moon on the Hill', Hill Road *(JDW)*
CP	SCILL, Robin Hood Lane *(Private)*
CP	Sutton Station, Platform *(Southern)*

Wallington	Beddington Park, Church Road (Daytime)
	Mellows Park (Daytime)
	'Whispering Moon', Woodcote Road *(JDW)*

Tower Hamlets

Bethnal Green	'Nandos', 366 Bethnal Green Road *(Nandos)*
Bow	Armagh Road Local Housing Office (Office hrs)
	Heylyn Square Local Housing Office (Office hrs)
	Thames Magistrates Court *(Courts Service)*
	'Bar Risa/Jongleurs', Bow Wharf *(Private)*
	'Match Maker', 580 Roman Road *(JDW)*
	'Morgan Arms', Morgan Street *(Private)*
Canary Wharf	Jubilee Place Mall *(Private)*
	'All Bar One', South Colonade *(M&B)*
	'Café Rouge', Mackenzie Walk *(Private)*
	'Cat & Canary', Fishermans Walk *(Fullers)*
	'Fine Line', Fishermans Walk *(Fullers)*
	'Nandos', Cabot Place East *(Nandos)*
	'Nandos', Jubilee Place *(Nandos)*
	'Pizza Express', Cabot Place East *(Private)*
	'Slug & Lettuce', South Colonnade *(Private)*
	'Wagamamas', Jubilee Place *(Private)*
Limehouse	'Oporto', West India Dock Rd *(Private)*
Mile End	'Half Moon', Mile End Road *(JDW)*
	'Hayfield', Mile End Road *(Private)*
	'Nandos', 9-25 Mile End Road *(Nandos)*
Poplar	East India Dock Road/Burdett Road
	Idea Store, East India Dock Road (Library hrs)
	Local Housing Office, Market Square
	'Gun', Coldharbour *(Private)*
Shoreditch	Shoreditch High Street Station *(London Overground)*
Wapping	'Cape', Thomas More Square *(Private)*
	'Prospect of Whitby', Wapping Wall *(Private)*
West India Quay	'Bar 38', Hertsmere Road *(Private)*
	'The Ledger Building', Hertsmere Road *(JDW)*
Whitechapel	Whitechapel Market
	Whitechapel Ideas Store (Library hrs)
	'Goodmans Fields', Mansell Street *(JDW)*

Waltham Forest

Chingford	Ridgeway Park, Old Church Road (Park hrs)
	Royal Hunting Lodge *(City of London)*
	Sainsbury's Store, Walthamstow Ave *(Sainsbury)*
	Chingford Station, off Platform 2 *(NX East Anglia)*
	'KFC', Albert Crescent *(KFC)*
	'King's Ford', Chingford Mount Road *(JDW)*
	'Kings Head', Kings Head Hill *(Private)*
	'The Obelisk', Old Church Road *(Private)*
	'Queen Elizabeth', Forest Side *(Private)*
	'Station House', Station Road *(Marstons)*
Leyton	Tesco Store, 825 High Road *(Tesco)*
	'Burger King', Leyton Mills *(Burger King)*
	'The Drum', 557 Lea Bridge Road *(JDW)*
	'KFC', Leyton Mills *(KFC)*
	Gala Bingo, Lea Bridge Road *(Gala)*
Leytonstone	Tesco Store, Leytonstone High Rd *(Tesco)*
	Leytonstone Bus Station, Church Road *(TfL)*
	'Heathcote Arms', 344 Grove Green Road *(Private)*
	'O'Neills', 762 High Road *(M&B)*
	'Walnut Tree', 857 High Road *(JDW)*
Walthamstow	The Mall Walthamstow *(Private)*
	Walthamstow Bus Station, Selborne Rd *(TfL)*
	'The Goose', 264 Hoe Street *(Private)*

Wandsworth

Balham	'Clarence', Balham High Road *(Private)*
	'Jackdaw & Rook', Balham High Rd *(Fullers)*
	'Moon Under Water', Balham High Rd *(JDW)*
Battersea	Station Approach, Clapham Junction
	Clapham Junction Station, Subway *(SW Trains)*
	'The Asparagus', Falcon Road *(JDW)*
	'Bank', Northcote Road *(Fullers)*
	'Duck', Battersea Rise *(Private)*
	'Falcon', St John's Hill *(Private)*
	'Nandos', Northcote Road *(Nandos)*
	'Northcote', Northcote Road *(Private)*
	'Prince Albert', Albert Bridge Road *(Private)*
	'Revolution', Lavender Hill *(Private)*

'Wakabout', Lavender Gardens *(Private)*

Putney	Putney Bridge Road/Putney High Street
	Putney Vale Cemetery (Cemetery hrs)
	Exchange Shopping Centre *(Private)*
	'Cedar Tree', Putney Bridge Road *(Private)*
	'Dukes Head', Lower Richmond Road *(Youngs)*
	'Old Spotted Horse', Putney High Street *(Youngs)*
	'The Railway', Upper Richmond Rd *(JDW)*
	'Real Greek Souvlaki', Putney High St *(Private)*
	'The Rocket', Putney Wharf Tower *(JDW)*
	'Slug & Lettuce', Putney High Street *(Private)*
Southfields	Earlsfield Library, Magdalen Rd (Library hrs)
	'Grid Inn', Replingham Road *(JDW)*
	'Old Garage', Replingham Road *(Greene King)*
	'Windmill Tea Rooms', Wimbledon Common *(Private)*
Tooting	Tooting Bec Common, Dr Johnson Avenue
	Tooting Bec Lido (Lido hrs)
	Tooting Broadway/Garratt Lane
	'A Bar 2 Far', Mitcham Road *(Private)*
	'J J Moons', Tooting High Street *(JDW)*
	'Kings Head', Upper Tooting Road *(Private)*
	'Leather Bottle', 538 Garratt Lane *(Youngs)*
	'McDonalds', Mitcham Road *(McDonalds)*
	'Mitre Hotel', Mitcham Road *(Private)*
	'Nandos', 224 Upper Tooting Rd *(Nandos)*
	'Tramshed', Mitcham Road *(Private)*
Wandsworth	Wandsworth High St, by Southside Centre
	'Alma', Old York Road *(Youngs)*
	'Nandos', Southside Shopping Centre *(Nandos)*
	'Queen Adelaide', Putney Bridge Road *(Private)*
	'Rose & Crown', Wandsworth High Street *(Private)*

Westminster (See also Central London)

Bayswater	'Nandos', 63 Westbourne Grove *(Nandos)*
Maida Vale	'Elgin Bar & Grill', Elgin Avenue *(Private)*
St Johns Wood	Salisbury Street/Church Street (7.30-18.00)
	Wellington Place, by Lords (10.00-18.00)
	Lords Cricket Ground (Matchdays) *(MCC)*

SOUTH EAST ENGLAND

Adur

Lancing	Beach Green
	Yew Tree Close, South Street
Lancing Beach	Shopsdam Road
	Widewater, West Beach Road
Shoreham Beach	Fort Haven
Shoreham-by-Sea	Adur Recreation Ground, Brighton Road
	Beach Green, Beach Road
	Buckingham Park
	Civic Centre, Ham Road
	Middle Street
Southwick	Southwick Beach, Basin Road (F only)
	Southwick Square (Mon-Sat)

Arun

Aldingbourne	Aldingbourne Counatry Centre (Centre hrs)
Aldwick	Marine Park Gardens
	West Park
Angmering	Haskins Roundstone Garden Centre *(Private)*
Arundel	Crown Yard
	Mill Road
Bognor Regis	Bedford Street (via steps)
	East Promenade Foreshore Office
	Hotham Park, High Street
	London Road Car Park
	Regis Centre
	Waterloo Square (via steps)
	Bognor Regis Station *(Southern)*
	'Hatters Inn', Queensway *(JDW)*
	Rowan Park Caravan Site *(Caravan Club)*
Felpham	Blakes Road
	'Southdowns', Felpham Way *(Private)*
Littlehampton	Arun Civic Centre (Office hrs)
	Coastguard Toilets
	Norfolk Gardens

	St Martins Car Park
	Littlehampton Station, Ticket Office *(Southern)*
	'George Inn', Surrey Street *(JDW)*
	Littlehampton Caravan Club Site *(Caravan Club)*
Middleton-on-Sea	Shrubbs Field
Pagham	Sandy Road
Rustington	Broadmark Avenue *(Parish Council)*
	Churchill Car Park *(Parish Council)*
	The Street, by Church *(Parish Council)*
	Woodlands Centre, Recreation Ground *(Parish Council)*

Ashford

Ashford	Bank Street
	Church Road
	Forge Lane, New Rents
	Park Street/North Street
	St Johns Lane
	County Mall Shopping Centre *(Private)*
	Sainsburys Store, Bybrook *(Sainsbury)*
	Waitrose Store, Templer Way *(Waitrose)*
	Ashford International Station, Platforms *(SE Rlwy)*
	'County Hotel', High Street *(JDW)*
	Ashford Bowl, Station Road *(AMF)*
Chilham	Taylors Hill Car Park
Tenterden	Recreation Ground Road
	St Michaels Recreation Ground
	Station Road
CP	Tenterden Gateway, High St (Office hrs)
Woodchurch	Front Road Car Park

Brighton & Hove

Aldrington	Recreation Ground, Saxon Rd (8.00-16.00, later in summer)
Brighton & Hove Seafront	Black Rock (Summer only, 9.30-18.00)
	King Alfred, Kings Esplanade (8.00-20.00, later in summer)
	Kings Esplanade, First Avenue (8.00-20.00, later in summer)
	Lagoon, Kingsway (8.00-17.00, later in summer)
	Lower Prom, E of Brighton Pier (Summer, 8.00-20.00)
	Lower Prom, West Street (8.00-18.00, later in summer)

CP   Madeira Drive, Colonnade (8.00-18.00, later in summer)
Madeira Drive, Play Area (10-17, later in summer)
Western Esplanade, Kingsway (8.00-17.00, later in summer)
Brighton Pier, by café *(Private)*
Concord 2, Madeira Hall *(Private)*
'Terraces Bar', Madeira Drive *(Private)*

Brighton Town Centre   Booth Museum, Dyke Road (Museum hrs)
Brighton History Centre, Church Street (Centre hrs)
Brighton Museum & Art Gallery (Museum hrs)
Jubilee Library, Church Street (Library hrs)
The Lanes, Black Lion Street (8.00-20.00, later in summer)
Old Steine (8.00-20.00, later in summer)
Prince Regent Swimming Complex (Centre hrs)
Providence Place, Car Park (8.00-20.00, later in summer)
Queens Park, West Drive (2) (10.00-20.00, later in summer)
Royal Pavilion (Opening hrs)
Royal Pavilion Gardens (M+F) (8.00-20.00, later in summer)
Brighton Law Courts *(Courts Service)*
'Bright Helm', West Street *(JDW)*
'Browns', Ship Street *(Private)*
'Browns Restaurant', Duke Street *(Private)*
'Caffe Nero', Prince Albert Street *(Private)*

'Curve Bar', Gardner Street *(Private)*
'Ha! Ha! Bar', Pavilion Buildings *(Private)*
'Nandos', 34 Duke Street *(Nandos)*
'Standard', West Street *(Private)*
'Varsity', East Street *(Barracuda)*
'Yates's Bar', West Street *(Yates)*
Duke of Yorks Cinema, Preston Circus *(Private)*

Brighton Marina	Mermaid Walk *(Private)* 'Karmer', Waterfront *(Private)* 'West Quay', Brighton Marina Village *(JDW)* BowlPlex *(Private)*
East Brighton	Blakers Park, Cleveland Road (10.00-18.00) Moulscombe Community Centre (Centre hrs) Patcham Library (Library hrs) Stanley Deeson Leisure Centre (Centre hrs) Stanmer Village (8.00-18.00, later in summer) Whitehawk Library (Library hrs) Wild Park (Summer and weekends, 9.00-18.00) Withdean Sports Centre (Centre hrs) Sheepcote Valley Caravan Park *(Caravan Club)*
Hangleton	Grenadier, Hangleton Road (8.00-20.00, later in summer) Hangleton Library, West Way (Library hrs)
Hove	Goldstone Villas/Eaton Villas (8.00-20.00, later in summer) Hove Cemetery, South Side (Cemetery hrs) Hove Library (Library hrs) Hove Museum & Art Gallery (Museum hrs) Hove Park (8.00-16.00, later in summer) Hove Recreation Ground (8.00-16.00, later in summer) Norton Road (8.00-20.00, later in summer) St Ann's Well Gardens (8.00-16.00, later in summer) West Blatchington Windmill (Business hrs) Hove Station, Platform *(Southern)* 'Station', Goldstone Villas *(Private)*
Kemptown	Gala Bingo, Freshfield Business Pk. *(Gala)*
Ovingdean	Undercliff (10.00-16.00, later in summer)
Portslade	Easthill Park (10.00-16.0, longer in summer) Foredown Tower (Business hrs) Mile Oak Library (Library hrs) Portslade Library (Library hrs)

	Station Road (8.00-20.00, later in summer)
	Victoria Recreation Ground (8.00-16.00, later in summer)
	Victoria Road (8.00-17.00)
Preston Park	Chalet (8.00-16.00, later in summer)
	Lawn Memorial Cemetery, Warren Road (Cemetery hrs)
	Preston Manor (Business hrs)
	Rotunda (8.00-16.00, later in summer)
Rottingdean	Rottingdean Recreation Ground (8.00-20.00, later in summer)
	Undercliff (7.00-20.00, later in summer)
Saltdean	Undercliff Walk (8.00-17.00, later in summer)

Canterbury

Canterbury	Best Lane
	Canterbury Lane
	City Council Offices, Military Road (Office hrs)
	Longport
	Pound Lane
	St Peter's Place
	Toddlers Cove (April-early October)
	Wincheap Park
	Worthgate
	BHS, Marlowe Arcade *(BHS)*
	Debenhams Store, Guildhall Sq *(Debenhams)*
	Sainsbury's Store, Kingsmead Rd *(Sainsbury)*
	Sidney Cooper Gallery, St Peters St *(Gallery hrs)*
	Canterbury East Station, Platform 2 *(SE Rlwy)*
	Canterbury West Station, Platform 1 *(SE Rlwy)*
	'Nandos', 46 St Peters Street *(Nandos)*
	'Thomas Ingoldsby', Burgate *(JDW)*
	'West Gate Inn', North Lane *(JDW)*
Fordwich	'George & Dragon', King Street *(Private)*
Herne Bay	Bandstand
	Beltinge
	Council Offices, William Street (Office hrs)
	Hampton Pier
	Hampton Pleasure Gardens (Easter-early Oct)
	Herne Bay Cemetery
	Herne Village, Cherry Orchard
	Kings Hall

	Market Street
	Pier Entrance
	Reculver Country Park
	St George's
	William Street
	Herne Bay Station, Platform 2 *(SE Rlwy)*
	'The Saxon Shore', Central Parade *(JDW)*
Upstreet	Grove Ferry Picnic Site *(Kent CC)*
Whitstable	Blue Anchor
	Faversham Road (Easter-early Oct)
	Harbour Street
	Horse Bridge
	Priest & Sow
	St Anne's
	St John's
	Skinners Alley
	Tankerton Beach
	Whitstable Station, Platform 1 *(SE Rlwy)*
	Whitstable Bowl, Tower Parade *(Private)*

Chichester

Bosham	Bosham Lane Car Park (Daytime)
Bracklesham Bay	Bracklesham Beach Car Park
	'Lively Lady', Stocks Lane *(Private)*
Chichester	Avenue de Chartres MSCP (Daytime)
	Cathedral Way (Daytime)
	East Pallant Car Park (Daytime)
	Little London (Daytime)
	Market Road Car Park (Daytime)
	Northgate Car Park (Daytime)
	Portfield Cemetery (F only) (Cemetery hrs)
	Priory Park (7.30-dusk)
	Tower Street (Daytime)
	Chichester Cathedral *(Cathedral)*
	Chichester Station, Platform 1 *(Southern)*
	'Chicago Rock Café', Chichester Gate *(Private)*
	'Dolphin & Anchor', West Street *(JDW)*
	'Gatehouse', Chichester Gate *(JDW)*
	'Globe Inn', Southgate *(Private)*

	'Nandos', Chichester Gate *(Nandos)* 'Slug & Lettuce', Southgate *(Private)* 'The Vestry', Southgate *(Private)*
Cobnor	Footpath Car Park *(Harbour Conservancy)*
East Wittering	Bracklesham Lane Car Park (Daytime) Kingfisher Parade (Daytime)
Fishbourne	Roman Palace, Car Park *(Private)* 'Bulls Head' *(Private)*
Goodwood	Goodwood Racecourse (4) *(Private)*
Midhurst	Grange Road Car Park (Daytime) North Street Car Park (Daytime) 'The Wheatsheaf', Wool Lane *(Private)*
Petworth	Town Centre Car Park (Daytime)
Selsey	East Beach Amenity Area (Daytime) Hillfield Road (Daytime) Lifeboat Station, Kingsway (Daytime)
Sidlesham	Pagham Nature Reserve *(W Sussex CC)*
West Itchenor	The Street (F only)

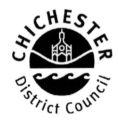

Chichester
District Council

For information on toilet facilities
and access to local attractions,
please visit our website
www.chichester.gov.uk
before you travel.

Alternatively please telephone
01243 785166

Best wishes from

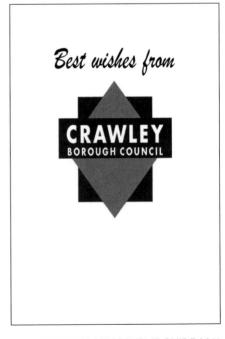

CRAWLEY
BOROUGH COUNCIL

West Wittering	Marine Drive Car Park (Daytime)
	Pound Road (Daytime)
	Pavillion Restaurant *(Private)*

Crawley

Bewbush	Dorsten Square
Broadfield	Broadfield Barton Car Park
	Buchan Country Park *(W Sussex CC)*
Crawley Town Centre	The Boulevard Car Park
	Bus Station, Friary Way
	Ifield Road, off High Street
	County Mall Shopping Centre *(Private)*
	Crawley Station, Platform 1 *(Southern)*
	'Bar Med', High Street *(Private)*
	'Coffee Republic', Queensway *(Private)*
	'Jubilee Oak', High Street *(JDW)*
	'Liquid Envy', Station Way *(Private)*
	'Nandos', Crawley Leisure Park *(Nandos)*
	'Rat & Parrot', High Street *(Private)*
	Longley Building *(Cent Sussex College)*
	Don Munro Block *(Cent Sussex College)*
	Crawley Bowl, Crawley Leisure Park *(AMF)*
Furnace Green	Weald Drive Parade
Gatwick	Gatwick Station, Platform 1 *(Network Rail)*
Gossops Green	Capel Lane Parade
Langley Green	Langley Drive Parade
Lowfield Heath	Amberley Fields Caravan Club Site *(Caravan Club)*
Maidenbower	Maidenbower Square
Northgate	Woodfield Road Parade
Pease Pottage	Pease Pottage Services A23 *(Moto)*
	'Black Swan', Old Brighton Road *(Private)*
	K2 Leisure Centre, Brighton Road *(Private)*
Pound Hill	Worth Road Parade
Three Bridges	Gales Drive, Gales Place
Tilgate	Ashdown Drive Parade
	Tilgate Park, Car Park

'Tilgate', Ashdown Drive *(Private)*

West Green — Snell Hatch Cemetery (Cemetery hrs)

Dartford

Bluewater — **CP** Bluewater Shopping Centre *(Private)*
House of Fraser Store *(Private)*
'Nando's', The Wintergarden *(Private)*

Dartford — Central Park, Cranford Street (Park hrs)
Dartford Civic Centre (Office hrs)
Hesketh Park (Park hrs)
Market Street, nr. Library (8.15-18.00)
Tree Community Centre, Cedar Rd (Centre hrs)
Orchards Shopping Centre *(Private)*
Priory Centre Car Park *(Private)*
Dartford Station, Booking Hall *(SE Rlwy)*
'Crush', Spital Street *(Private)*
'Flying Boat', Spital Street *(JDW)*
'Litten Tree', Spital Street *(Private)*
'Paper Moon', High Street *(JDW)*
'Royal Victoria & Bull', High Street *(Private)*
'Tollgate', High Street *(Private)*
Gala Bingo, Spital Street *(Gala)*

Greenhithe — Greenhithe Station, Platform 2 *(SE Rlwy)*

Longfield — Waitrose Car Park *(Private)*

Dover

Ash — Village Car Park, The Street

Deal — Deal Pier
King Street
Kingsdown Road/Granville Road
Town Hall
Deal Station, Waiting Room *(SE Rlwy)*

Dover — Buckland Bridge
The Clock Tower
CP Dover Gateway, Castle Street (Office hrs)
East Cliff
Kearsney Abbey
Maison Dieu Gardens
Stembrook Car Park

	White Cliffs Visitor Centre *(Nat. Trust)*
	Charlton Shopping Centre *(Private)*
	Dover Priory Station, Waiting Room *(SE Rlwy)*
	'Eight Bells', Cannon Street *(JDW)*
	'Millers', Marine Parade *(Private)*
	Gala Bingo, Biggin Street *(Gala)*
Sandwich	The Quay
St Margarets at Cliffe	St Margarets Bay
Wingham	Village Car Park

Eastbourne

Beachy Head	Beachy Head Car Park
Eastbourne	The Archery, Channel View Road
	Bandstand, Upper Promenade (M+F)
	Bandstand, Lower Promenade
	Coach Station, Junction Road
	Devonshire Park, Congress Car Park (2)
	Fishermen's Green
	Helen Gardens, rear of Pavilion
	Holywell, Lower Promenade

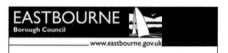

Hyde Gardens, by Tourist Information Centre
Pier, Lower Promenade
Princes Park, by Café
Redoubt, by Bowls Pavilion
Wartling Road
Arndale Shopping Centre (3) *(Private)*
Enterprise Shopping Centre, Car Park *(Private)*
Eastbourne Station, Concourse *(Southern)*
'The Lamb', Old Town *(Harveys)*
'London & County', Terminus Road *(JDW)*
'The Terminus', Terminus Road *(Harveys)*
'Wetherspoons', Cornfield Road *(JDW)*
Aldro Building, Darley Road *(Univ of Brighton)*
Queenswood, Darley Road *(Univ of Brighton)*
Stiokers, Carlisle Road *(Univ of Brighton)*

Hampden Park	Hampden Park, by Cafe
Langney	Langney Point, Car Park
	Langney Shopping Centre Car Park *(Private)*
South Harbour	The Waterfront, nr. Pedestrian entrance

Elmbridge

Claygate	Recreation Ground, Church Road (Daytime)
Cobham	Hollyhedge Road
	'Brasserie Gerard', Oakdene Parade *(Private)*
East Molesey	Molesey Lock, Hurst Road
	Walton Road Car Park
	Hampton Court Station *(SW Trains)*
	'Prince of Wales', Bridge Road *(Greene King)*
Esher	High Street
	'Marquis of Granby', Portsmouth Rd *(Private)*
	Sandown Park Racecourse (Racedays) *(Private)*
Hersham	Hersham Green Shopping Centre *(Private)*
Walton-on-Thames	Cowey Sale Car Park, Walton Bridge
	Walton Library, The Heart (Library hrs) *(Surrey CC)*
	'Ashley Park', Ashley Park Road *(Private)*
	'Nandos', 7 The Heart *(Nandos)*
	'The Regent', Church Street *(JDW)*
	'Wagamama' The Heart *(Private)*

West Molesey	Recreation Ground, Walton Road
Weybridge	Churchfield Road (Daytime)
	High Street, behind shops
	Weybridge Station, Platform 1 *(SW Trains)*
	'Slug & Lettuce', High Street *(Private)*
	Brooklands Museum *(Private)*

Epsom & Ewell

Epsom	Alexandra Recreation Ground (Daytime)
	Ashley Road Cemetery (Cemetery hrs)
	Ebbisham Centre (Centre hrs)
	Epsom Town Hall (Office hrs)
	Horton Country Park, Horton Lane (Daytime)
	The Mall Ashley *(Private)*
	'Assembly Rooms', High Street *(JDW)*
	'Nandos', The Oaks Square *(Nandos)*
	'Yates's Bar', Derby Square *(Yates)*
Epsom Downs	Tattenham Corner (Daytime)
Ewell	Bourne Hall (Hall hrs)

Gravesham

Ebbsfleet	Ebbsfleet Station, Concourse *(SE Rlwy)*
Gravesend	Anglesea Shopping Centre, Clive Road
	Borough Market, Queen Street
	Gordon Promenade
	St George's Centre (Shopping hrs)
	Visitor Centre, St Georges Square (Centre hrs)

	Woodlands Park, Dashwood Road [Temp closed] Debenhams Store, New Road *(Debenhams)* Gravesend Station, Platform 1 *(SE Rlwy)* 'Pembroke', King Street *(Barracuda)* 'Robert Pocock', Windmill Street *(JDW)*
Higham	School Lane
Meopham	Camer Park, Camer Park Road Wrotham Road/Pitfield Drive

Guildford

Ash Common	Recreation Ground *(Parish Council)*
Burpham	Sutherland Memorial Park (Park hrs)
Guildford	Allen House, by York Road MSCP (7.00-19.00) Bedford Road Car Park {Closed at present] Farnham Road MSCP (7.00-19.00) Shalford Park, Shalford Road (7.00-19.00) Stoke Park, by Nurseries (7.00-19.00) Stoke Park, by Challenger Centre (7.00-17.00) Stoke Park, Tennis Courts (7.00-17.00) Tunsgate, Guildford High Street (7.30-19.00) Ward Street (7.30-19.00) Woodbridge Road (7.00-19.00) Debenhams Store, Millbrook *(Debenhams)* Guildford Station, Platform 2 *(SW Trains)* 'George Abbot', High Street/Riverside *(Private)* 'Ha! Ha! Bar', North Street *(Private)* 'Nandos', Friary Street *(Nandos)* 'Old Orleans', Wayside Square *(Private)* 'Rodboro Buildings', Bridge Street *(JDW)* 'Stoke', Stoke Road *(Private)*
Ripley	High Street
Shere	Middle Street *(Parish Council)*

Hastings

Hastings	Alexandra Park, Tennis Pavilion Hastings Country Park, Coastguard Lane Hastings Country Park, Helipad Rock a Nore Road Hastings Station, Ticket Hall *(SE Rlwy)*

	'John Logie Baird', Havelock Road *(JDW)* 'Yates's Bar', Robertson Street *(Yates)*
Ore	Ore Village, Fairlight Road
St Leonards	Warrior Square 'Royal Hotel' *(Private)*

Horsham

Amberley	Chalk Pits (Daytime) Houghton Bridge Tea Garden (Daytime)
Billingshurst	Mill Lane Car Park
Bramber	The Street Car Park
Dial Post	Honeybridge Caravan Park *(Private)*
Henfield	High Street Car Park
Horsham	The Forum, Lower Tanbridge Way (Daytime) North Parade Boxing Club (Club hrs) Piries Place Car Park (Daytime) Swan Walk Shopping Centre *(Private)* 'Green Dragon', Bishopric *(Private)* 'Lynd Cross', Springfield Road *(JDW)*
Southwater	Southwater Country Park (Park hrs)
Steyning	High Street Car Park Steyning Centre
Washington	Village Hall

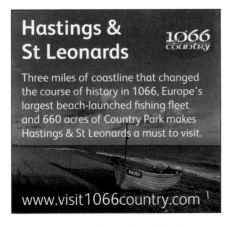

Lewes

Ditchling	Village Hall Car Park
Glynde	Recreation Ground
Lewes	Greyfriars
	Market Lane
	Southover Grange Gardens (8.00-dusk)
	Western Road
	'The Dorset', Malling Street *(Harveys)*
Newhaven	Fort Road
	Lower Place
	Newhaven Fort
Peacehaven	Meridian Centre (9.00-17.00)
	Peacehaven Leisure Centre
	Roderick Avenue
Ringmer	Village Hall
Seaford	The Buckle
	Martello Tower
	Place Lane
	Salts Recreation Ground

Maidstone

Allington	Mid Kent Shopping Centre (8.30-18.00)
Aylesford	Cobtree Park, Ranger Centre (7.00-16.30)
Bearsted	Bearsted Caravan Club Site *(Caravan Club)*
Headcorn	Kings Road, Days Green (7.00-21.00)
	Headcorn Station, Platform 2 *(SE Rlwy)*
Lenham	Maidstone Road (7.00-18.00)
Maidstone	Brenchley Gardens (M+F) (Daytime)
	Clare Park, Tonbridge Road (Park hrs)
	Corn Exchange, Market Buildings (7.00-21.00)
	Fairmeadow (7.00-20.00)
	Lockmeadow Market Centre (7.00-16.00)
	Mote Park (2) (7.00-18.00)
	Penenden Heath Road
	South Park (7.00-18.00)
	Whatman Park (8.00-16.00)
	Fremlin Walk, Earl Street *(Private)*

Fremlin Walk, off Week Street *(Private)*
The Mall Chequers, by Bus Station *(Private)*
Royal Star Arcade *(Private)*
Maidstone East Station, Platform 1 *(SE Rlwy)*
'Caffe Nero', King Street *(Private)*
'Chicago Rock Café', High Street *(Private)*
'J.J's', Lockmeadow Entertainment Centre *(Private)*
'Liquid', Lockmeadow Entertainment Centre *(Private)*
'Muggleton Inn', High Street *(JDW)*
'Nandos', 29 Earl Street *(Nandos)*
'Society Rooms', Week Street *(JDW)*
'Zebra Bar', King Street *(Private)*
Gala Bingo, Lower Stone Street *(Gala)*
Maidstone Bowl, King Street *(AMF)*
CP Maidstone Gateway, King Street (Office hrs)

Marden	High Street, Library Car Park (7.00-21.00)
Staplehurst	Bell Lane (7.00-18.00) Staplehurst Shopping Parade (7.00-17.00) Stapplehurst Station, Platform 1 *(SE Rllwy)*
Sutton Valence	North Street, by Village Hall (6.00-18.00)
Yalding	The Lees

Medway

Chatham	Capstone Farm Country Park Luton Recreation Ground, Capstone Road (Matchdays) Chatham Station, Platform 2 *(SE Rlwy)* 'Nandos', Dickens World *(Nandos)* 'Old Ash Tree', Rainham Road *(Private)* Gala Bingo, High Street *(Gala)*
Cliffe	The Buttway (8.00-18.00)
Gillingham	Canterbury Street (M+F) (8.00-18.00) Sappers Walk, High Street Riverside Country Park Strand, Pier Road (8.00-18.00, later in summer) Gillingham Station, Platformas 1/2 & 3 *(SE Rlwy)* Priestfield Stadium (7) (Matchdays) *(Private)*
Hempstead	Hempstead Valley Centre (2) *(Private)*
Hoo	Stoke Road

Lower Upnor	The Waterfront
Parkwood	Parkwood Green (8.00-18.00)
Rainham	Shopping Precinct, Longley Rd (8.00-18.00)
	Rainham Station, Platform 1 *(SE Rlwy)*
Rainham M2	Medway Services, Juncts 4/5 *(Moto)*
Rochester	Acorn Wharf Coach Park (8.00-18.00, later in summer)
	Castle Gardens (8.00-18.00, later in summer)
	Northgate (8.00-18.00, later in summer)
	'Golden Lion', High Street *(JDW)*
Strood	Newark Yard
	'McDonalds', Commercial Road *(McDonalds)*
	Gala Bingo, Chariot Way *(Gala)*
Twydall Green	Shopping Centre (M+F) (8.00-15.00)
Walderslade	'Sherwood Oak', Robin Hood Lane *(Private)*

Mid Sussex

Ardingly	High Street *(Parish Council)*
Burgess Hill	Janes Lane Recreation Ground Pavilion
	The Martlets Shopping Centre, by Library
	St Johns Park
Cuckfield	Cuckfield Recreation Ground (April-Sept)
	Broad Street Car Park *(Parish Council)*
Devils Dyke	by Devils Dyke Hotel *(Private)*
East Grinstead	King Street Car Park
	Mount Noddy Recreation Ground

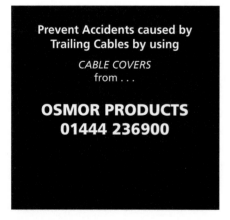

	'Caffe Nero', High Street *(Private)* 'Old Mill', Dunnings Road *(Harveys)* 'Ounce & Ivy Bush', The Atrium *(JDW)*
Handcross	'Red Lion', High Street *(Private)*
Hassocks	Adastra Park, Keymer Road
Haywards Heath	The Orchards Shopping Centre Car Park Victoria Park, South Road 'The Heath', Sussex Road *(Harveys)*
Lindfield	Denmans Lane Car Park *(Parish Council)*

Mole Valley

Ashtead	Memorial Car Park, off High Street
Bookham	Lower Shott Car Park off A246
Box Hill	A24, Car Park opp. Burford Bridge Hotel *(Surrey CC)*
Dorking	St Martins Walk, Church Square *(Private)*
Leatherhead	Swan Shopping Centre Leatherhead Station *(Southern)* 'Edmund Tylney', High Street *(JDW)* 'Penny Black', North Street *(Youngs)*

Reigate & Banstead

Banstead	High Street Car Park (8.00-19.00) Lady Neville Recreation Park (8.00-19.00) 'The Woolpack' *(Private)*
Earlswood	Earlswood Lakes, Woodhatch Road (7.30-17.00)

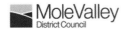

MoleValley
District Council

For more information on
Public Facilities and access to many
attractions why not telephone for
more details before you travel?

Please telephone for all enquiries:

01306 885 001

Reigate & Banstead
BOROUGH COUNCIL
Banstead I Horley I Redhill I Reigate

For more information telephone
our Council Helpline on
01737 27600

Banstead
High Street Car Park
Lady Neville Recreation Ground
'The Woolpack' PH (Private)
Earlswood Earlswood Lakes, Woodhatch Road
Horley Consort Way
Redhill
Station Road, by McDonalds
opp Bus Station (Private)
Reigate
Bell Street, by Supermarket
Reigate Hill, Car Park

Horley	Consort Way
	'Jack Fairman', Victoria Road *(JDW)*
Merstham	Aldersted Heath Caravan Club Site *(Caravan Club)*
Redhill	Station Road, by McDonalds
	'The Sun', London Road *(JDW)*
Reigate	Bell Street, by supermarket (8.00-19.00)
Walton-on-the Hill	'The Chequers', Chequers Road *(Youngs)*

Rother

Battle	Mount Street Car Park
	Normanhurst Court Caravan Site *(Caravan Club)*
Bexhill	Bexhill Cemetery
	Channel View East
	Cooden Sea Road
	Devonshire Road
	East Parade
	Egerton Park
	Little Common Recreation Ground
	Little Common Roundabout

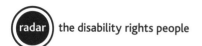

the disability rights people

Become a member of Radar

Network with like-minded people and keep up to date with disability sector news.

www.radar.org.uk

For more information on public facilities, why not telephone for more details before you travel?

Please telephone for all enquiries:

Rother
District Council

01424 787 000

	Manor Barn, by Car Park
	Normans Bay (Easter to October)
	Polegrove Grandstand
	Sidley
	West Parade
Burwash	Car Park
Camber	Central Car Park (Easter-October)
	West Car Park (Easter-October)
Iden	Village Hall *(Hall Committee)*
Pett	Pett Level Car Park
	Fairlight Wood Caravan Park *(Caravan Club)*
Robertsbridge	Car Park
Rye	Gun Gardens
	Lucknow Place
	Rye Harbour
	Station Approach, Crownfield
	The Strand
Sedlescombe	Car Park
Ticehurst	Village
Winchelsea	Winchelsea Town
	Winchelsea Beach (Summer)

Runnymede

Chertsey	off Guildford Street

Sevenoaks

Edenbridge	Market Yard Car Park *(Town Council)*
Farningham	'Pied Bull', High Street *(Private)*
Horton Kirby	Westminster Field, The Street *(Parish Council)*
Ide Hill	Wheatsheaf Hill
	'Woodman', Whitley Row *(Private)*
Kemsing	St Edith's Hall, High Street
Leigh	Crandells
Otford	High Street *(Parish Council)*
Penshurst	High Street

Riverhead	'Bullfinch' *(Private)*
Sevenoaks	Bus Station, High Street
	Lower St Johns Car Park *(Town Council)*
	The Vine Gardens *(Town Council)*
	Sevenoaks Station, Concourse *(SE Rlwy)*
	'Oak Tree', High Street *(Barracuda)*
	'The Sennockian', High Street *(JDW)*
Shoreham	Rangers Lodge, St Andrews Wood
	High Street *(Parish Council)*
Sundridge	'White Horse', Main Street *(Private)*
Swanley	Station Road
	Swanley Park, New Barn Rd *(Town Council)*
Westerham	Fullers Hill *(Parish Council)*

Shepway

Cheriton	Somerset Road
Densole	Blackhorse Farm Caravan Club Site *(Caravan Club)*
Dymchurch	High Street
Folkestone	Leas Cliff Hall, The Leas
	Pleydell Gardens
	Radnor Park, Cheriton Road
	Roman Remains, East Cliff (Summer)
	The Stade, Folkestone Harbour
	Sunny Sands, Coronation Parade (Summer)
	Toll Gate, Lower Sandgate Road
	Folkestone Central Station, Booking Hall *(SE Rlwy)*
	'Samuel Peto', Rendezvous St *(JDW)*
Greatstone	Jolly Fisherman, Coast Drive
Hythe	Chapel Street
	Cinque Ports, Stade Street
	Marine Parade, Saltwood Gardens (Summer)
	Prospect Road
Lydd	Coronation Square
	Lade Car Park
New Romney	Car Park, Church Road
St Marys Bay	High Knocke Car Park

| West Hythe | Daleacres Caravan Club Site *(Caravan Club)* |

Spelthorne

Ashford	Church Road, by MSCP
	'Royal Hart', Church Road *(Private)*
Laleham	Laleham Park, Pavilion Kiosk
Shepperton	High Street
	Shepperton Locks, Towpath
Staines	Memorial Gardens, opp Debenhams
	Elmsleigh Shopping Centre (2) *(Private)*
	'Blue Anchor', High Street *(Private)*
	'The George', High Street *(JDW)*
	'Nandos', Two Rives *(Nandos)*
	'Que Pasa', Tillys Lane *(Marstons)*
Sunbury	Walled Garden
	Sunbury Cross Shopping Centre *(Private)*

Surrey Heath

Bagshot	Park Street
Camberley	Knoll Road by MSCP, behind Theatre
	Martindale Avenue, Heatherside
	Watchetts Park (Daytime)
	The Mall Main Square *(Private)*
	'Claude Du Vall', High Street *(JDW)*
	'Que Pasa', High Street *(Marstons)*
	'Yates's Bar', High Street *(Yates)*
	BowlPlex, The Atrium *(BowlPlex)*
Chobham	Car Park, off High Street
Frimley	Church Road
	Frimley Green Recreation Ground (Daytime)
	Frimley Lodge Park, Sturt Road (M+F)
Lightwater	Lightwater Country Park (Daytime)

Swale

Boughton	The Street/School Lane (Mon-Sat, daytime)
Faversham	Central Car Park
	Co-op Supermarket, South Road *(Co-op)*
	Faversham Station, Platform 1/2 (SE Rlwy)

	'The Leading Light', Preston Street *(JDW)*
Leysdown-on-Sea	The Grove (Seasonal, daytime)
	The Spinney, Leysdown Road
Minster	White House, the Broadway
Queenborough	Queenborough Park
Sheerness	Bridge Street
	Rose Street (Mon-Sat)
	Tesco Store, Bridge Road *(Tesco)*
Sittingbourne	Central Avenue
	The Forum (Mon-Sat)
	Sittingbourne Station *(SE Rlwy)*
	Asda Store *(Asda)*
	'The Summoner', High Street *(JDW)*

Tandridge

Bletchingley	'Millers', High Street *(Private)*
Burstow	'Shipley Bridge', Antlands Lane *(Private)*
Caterham	West Way/Chaldon Road
	'Pilgrim', Godstone Road *(Private)*
Dormansland	Dormans High Street
Godstone	A22 Southbound Lay-by, Godstone Hill
	Godstone Green
Lingfield	Godstone Road/Jenny Lane
Oxted	A25 Westbound, Nags Hall lay-by
	Ellice Road Car Park
	Station Road West
	Oxted Station *(Southern)*
	'Oxted Inn', Station Road West *(JDW)*
Warlingham	Leas Road/Westhall Road
Whyteleafe	Recreation Ground, Hillbury Road
	Station Road Car Park

Thanet

Birchington	Alpha Road Car Park (Daytime)
	Minnis Bay Car Park (Daytime)
Broadstairs	Clock Tower, Victoria Promenade (Daytime)

Croft's Place Car Park (Daytime)
Harbour (Daytime)
Hopeville Avenue, St Peters (Daytime)
Joss Bay (Summer, Daytime)
Broadstairs Station, Platform 1 *(SE Rlwy)*
'Captain Digby', Whiteness Road *(Private)*
'Nandos', Westwood Cross *(Nandos)*
G Casino, Westwood Cross *(Private)*
Mecca Bingo, Westwood Cross *(Mecca)*

Cliftonville   'Wheatsheaf', Northdown Park Rd *(Greene King)*

Margate   Buenos Ayres, Marine Terrace (Daytime)
The Centre Shopping Mall (Daytime)
College Walk Shopping Mall (Daytime)
Harbour Arm (Daytime)
Harold Road (Daytime)
The Oval Bandstand (Daytime)
CP Thanet Gateway, Cecil Street (Office hrs)
West Bay Promenade (Daytime)
Margate Station, Platform 1 *(SE Rlwy)*
Margate Magistrates Court *(Courts Service)*
'McDonalds', High Street *(McDonalds)*

Minster   High Street Car Park (Daytime)

Ramsgate   Bathing Station, Marina Esplanade (Summer, daytime)
Cavendish Street (Daytime)
East Pier Yard, Harbour (Daytime)
King George VI Park (Park hrs)
Marina Esplanade (Daytime)

Thanet District Council

Are pleased to support Radar

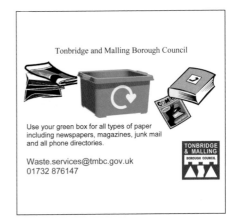

Tonbridge and Malling Borough Council

Use your green box for all types of paper including newspapers, magazines, junk mail and all phone directories.

Waste.services@tmbc.gov.uk
01732 876147

TONBRIDGE
& MALLING
BOROUGH COUNCIL

Screaming Alley, off Grange Road (Daytime)
Ramsgate Station, Concourse *(SE Rlwy)*
'Lounge Bar', Harbour Parade *(Private)*
'McDonalds', King Street *(McDonalds)*
'Sovereign', Harbour Street *(Private)*

| Westgate | St Mildred's Bay (Daytime) |
| | Station Road (Daytime) |

Tonbridge & Malling

Borough Green	High Street, Village Hall Car Park (6.00-18.00)
East Peckham	The Pound, Snoll Hatch Road (6.00-18.00)
Hadlow	Court Lane, A26 junction (6.00-18.00)
	'Two Brewers', Maidstone Road *(Harveys)*
Larkfield	Leybourne Country Park (Park hrs)
	Martin Square
Snodland	Rockfort Road, Car Park (6.00-18.00)
Tonbridge	Angel Centre (6.00-18.00)
	Castle Street (6.00-18.00)
	Haysden Country Park (Park hrs)
	Lamberts Yard, off High Street (6.00-18.00)
	Priory Road
	Racecourse Sports Ground (6.00-18.00)
CP	Tonbridge Gateway, Castle St (Office hrs)
	Tonbridge Station, Platform 3 *(SE Rlwy)*
	'Humphrey Bean', High Street *(JDW)*
	'Vauxhall Inn', Vauxhall Lane *(Private)*
West Malling	King Street, off High Street
	West Malling Station, Platform 1 *(SE Rlwy)*
Wrotham	High Street (6.00-18.00)

Tunbridge Wells

Cranbrook	Crane Lane (7.00-18.00)
	'White Horse', Carriers Road *(Private)*
Goudhurst	Balcombes Hill Car Park (7.00-18.00)
	Bedgebury National Pinetum *(Forest Enterprise)*
Hawkhurst	Kino Cinema, Rye Road (9.00-23.00) *(Private)*
Paddock Wood	Commercial Road Car Park East

Southborough	London Road, by Silk Restaurant (7.00-18.00)
	Pennington Grounds, Pennington Road
Sissinghurst	The Street (7.00-18.00)
Tunbridge Wells	Calverley Park (Park hrs)
	Camden Centre, Market Square (Centre hrs)
	Crescent Road Car Park/ (8.00-18.00, less Sundays)
	Dunorlan Park (Park hrs)
	Grosvenor Recreation Ground (Park hrs)
	Hawkenbury Recreation Ground (Park hrs)
	Kent & Sussex Cemetery (Cemetery hrs)
	St John's Recreation Ground Pavilion Park hrs)
CP	Tunbridge Wells Gateway, Grosvenor Rd (Office hrs)
	Union House, nr. Pantiles (7.00-18.00)
	Wellington Rocks, The Common (7.00-18.00)
	Corn Exchange, Pantiles *(Private)*
	Royal Victoria Place, nr. Shopmobility *(Private)*
	Sainsbury's Store, Linden Park Road *(Sainsbury)*
	Tunbridge Wells Station, Platform 1 *(SE Rlwy)*
	'Beau Nash', Mount Ephraim *(Private)*
	'Gourmet Burger Kitchen', Mount Pleasant Rd *(Private)*
	'Opera House', Mount Pleasant Road *(JDW)*
	'Robin Hood', Sandhurst Road *(Private)*
	'Wagamama', Mount Pleasant Road *(Private)*

Waverley

Bramley	Windrush Close
Cranleigh	Cricket Green, Guildford Road
	Village Way Car Park
Farncombe	Broadwater Park, Summers Road
	North Street
Farnham	Central Car Park, Victoria Road *(Town Council)*
	Farnham Station, Platform 1 *(SW Trains)*
Frensham	Frensham Great Pond Visitor Centre
Godalming	Crown Court, High Street
	Meadrow
	Winkworth Arboretum, by tearoom *(National Trust)*
	'Jack Phillips', High Street *(JDW)*
Haslemere	High Street Car Park

	Haslemere Station, Platform 2 *(SW Trains)*
	'Swan Inn', High Street *(JDW)*
Tilford	Tilford Green (April-Sept)
Witley	Witley Common Centre *(National Trust)*

Wealden

Alfriston	The Dene Car Park
	The Willows Car Park
Birling Gap	Car Park *(National Trust)*
Crowborough	Council Offices (Office hrs)
	Croft Road Car Park [Closed at present]
East Hoathly	'Foresters Arms', South Street *(Harveys)*
Forest Row	Lower Road Car Park (8.00-18.00)
Hailsham	Council Offices (Office hrs)
	Vicarage Field (Mon-Sat 8.00-18.00)
	St Marys Walk *(Private)*
	'George Hotel', George Street *(JDW)*
Heathfield	Station Road Car Park
Isfield	'Halfway House', Rose Hill *(Harveys)*
Mayfield	South Street Car Park
Pevensey	Pevensey Castle Car Park
Pevensey Bay	Sea Road (8.00-18.00)
Polegate	High Street

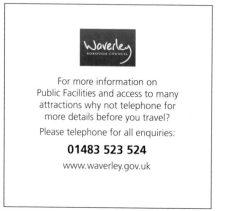

For more information on
Public Facilities and access to many
attractions why not telephone for
more details before you travel?

Please telephone for all enquiries:

01483 523 524

www.waverley.gov.uk

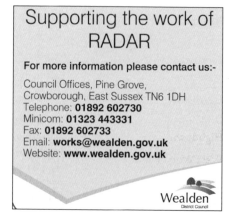

Supporting the work of RADAR

For more information please contact us:-

Council Offices, Pine Grove,
Crowborough, East Sussex TN6 1DH
Telephone: **01892 602730**
Minicom: **01323 443331**
Fax: **01892 602733**
Email: **works@wealden.gov.uk**
Website: **www.wealden.gov.uk**

Wealden
District Council

NATIONAL KEY SCHEME GUIDE 2011

Stone Cross	Glyndley Garden Centre *(Private)*
Uckfield	Luxford Field Car Park
	Tesco Store, Bell Farm Road *(Tesco)*
	Uckfield Bus Station *(Private)*
Wadhurst	Commemoration Hall, High St (8.00-18.00)
Willingdon	The Triangle, A22

Woking

Byfleet	Recreation Ground, Stream Close (Daytime)
Horsell	Wheatsheaf Common, Chobham Rd (Daytime)
Knaphill	High Street (Daytime)
	Knaphill Library (Library hrs) *(Surrey CC)*
Mayford	Mayford Village Hall (Hall hrs) *(Private)*
Sheerwater	Recreation Ground, Blackmore Cres (Daytime)
West Byfleet	Lavender Road (Daytime)
	'Claremont', Station Road *(Private)*
Woking	Addison Road (Daytime)
	Heathside Car Park (Mon-Sat, daytime)
	Market Square (Daytime)
	Victoria Way Car Park (Daytime)
	Woking Station, Platforms 1 & 4/5 *(SW Trains)*
	'Café Giardino', Wolsey Walk *(Private)*
	'Caffe Nero', Commercial Way *(Caffe Nero)*
	'Herbert Wells', Chertsey Road *(JDW)*
	'KFC', Chertsey Road *(KFC)*
	'O'Neills', Crown Square *(M&B)*
	'Rat & Parrot', Chertsey Road *(Private)*
	'RSVP', Chertsey Road *(Private)*
	'Station', Chertsey Road *(Private)*
	'Wheatsheaf', Chobham Road *(Private)*
	'Yates's Bar', Chobham Road *(Yates)*

Worthing

Highdown	Highdown Gardens, A259 (Daytime)
West Worthing	George V Avenue, by Post Office (Daytime)
Worthing	Beach House Park, Bowls Pavilion (Daytime)
	Buckingham Road (Daytime)

Homefield Park (Summer, Daytime)
Marine Gardens, nr. Café (Daytime)
Pier (Summer, Daytime)
Promenade by Lido, (Daytime)
Promenade, opp Dome (Daytime)
Sea Lane Car Park (Daytime)
Victoria Park (Daytime)
High Street MSCP *(NCP)*
Worthing Station *(Southern)*
'Caffe Nero', South Street *(Private)*
'Sir Timothy Shelley', Chapel Road *(JDW)*
'Que Pasa', Chapel Road *(Marstons)*
'Three Fishes', Chapel Road *(JDW)*
Gala Bingo, Rowlands Road *(Gala)*

Aylesbury Vale

Aston Clinton	'Duck Inn', London Road *(Private)*
Aylesbury	Anchor Lane Car Park (7.00-19.30)
	Cemetery (Cemetery hrs)
	Civic Centre MSCP
	Friarscroft Car Park (8.30-19.30)
	Upper Hundreds Car Park (7.30-19.30)
	Vale Park (7.30-19.30)
	Aylesbury Bus Station, Friars Square *(Private)*
	Aylesbury Station, Platform 3 *(Chiltern Railways)*
	'Bell Hotel', Market Square *(JDW)*
	'Chicago Rock Café', Exchange Street *(Private)*
	'Cotton Wheel', Jasckson Road *(Private)*
	'The Harrow', Cambridge Street *(Private)*
	'Litten Tree', Kingsbury Court *(Private)*
	'New Zealand', Buckingham Road *(Private)*
	'Slug & Lettuce', Exchange Street *(Private)*
	'Weavers', Park Street *(Private)*
	'White Hart', Exchange Street *(JDW)*
Bedgrove	'Buckinghamshire Yeoman', Cambourne Ave *(Private)*
Buckingham	Moreton Road (7.30-22.00)
	Swan Pool & Leisure Centre *(Private)*
Grove	'Grove Lock' *(Fullers)*
Stoke Mandeville	Bucks CC Sports & Social Club *(Private)*
Swanbourne	'Betsey Wynne', Mursley Road *(Private)*
Waddesdon	A41 Layby
Wendover	Library Car Park (7.30-19.30)
	Ellesborough Golf Club, Butlers Cross *(Private)*
Winslow	Greyhound Lane, Car Park (8.00-17.00)

Basingstoke & Deane

Basingstoke	Castons Yard, off New Road
	Eastrop Park
	New Road, by Red Lion Lane

	Worting Road Cemetery
CP	Basingstoke Discovery Centre (Hants CC)
	Potter's Walk, opp. Library *(Private)*
	Debenhams Store, Festival Pl *(Debenhams)*
	Viables Craft Centre, Harrow Way *(Private)*
	Basingstoke Station, Platforms 2/3 *(SW Trains)*
	'Lloyds Bar', Festival Place *(JDW)*
	'Maidenhead Inn', Winchester Street *(JDW)*
	'Nandos', Festival Place *(Nandos)*
	Gala Bingo, Basingstoke Leisure Pk. *(Gala)*
Kempshott	Old Down Close
	Stratton Park, by Pavilion
Kingsclere	Swan Street
Overton	Winchester Street, Community Car Park
St Mary Bourne	Bourne Meadow, opp. Village Hall
Tadley	Mulfords Hill
Whitchurch	Bell Street, Car Park

Bracknell Forest

Birch Hill	Birch Hill Shopping Parade, Leppington
Bracknell	Brooke House, High Street
	Bus Station, The Ring
	High Street MSCP, Level 4 (Daytime)
	Bracknell Station, Platform 1 *(SW Trains)*
	'Old Manor', Church Road *(JDW)*
	Hollywood Bowl, The Point *(AMF)*
Crowthorne	Napier Road, High Street
Warfield	'Shepherds House', Moss End *(Private)*

Cherwell

Ardley M40	Cherwell Valley Services, J10 M40 *(Moto)*
Banbury	Bridge Street, by Town Hall (6.00-19.00)
	Bus Station
	Horsefair (6.00-19.00)
	Hardwick Hill Cemetery (Daytime) *(Town Council)*
	Southam Rd Cemetery (Daytime) *(Town Council)*
	Debenhams Store, Castle Quay *(Debenhams)*

	Banbury Station, upper level *(Chiltern Railways)* 'The Exchange', High Street *(JDW)* 'Fleur-de-Lis', Broad Street *(JDW)* 'Que Pasa', High Street *(Marstons)*
Bicester	Bure Place, Crown Car Park (6.00-19.00) Claremont (6.00-19.00) 'Litten Tree', Sheep Street *(Private)* 'Penny Black', Sheep Street *(JDW)*
Kidlington	Watts Way Car Park, off High St (6.00-19.00)

Chiltern

Amersham on the Hill	Woodside Close, off Sycamore Rd (Daytime)
Chalfont St Giles	High Street (Daytime)
Chalfont St Peter	High Street
Chesham	Star Yard Car Park (Daytime) Lowndes Park *(Town Council)*
Great Missenden	Link Road (Daytime)
Little Chalfont	Snells Wood Car Park (Daytime)
Old Amersham	Dovecote Meadow, Car Park (Daytime)
Prestwood	High Street, Car Park (Daytime)

East Hampshire

Alton	CP	Lady Place Car Park Turk Street, Draymans Way Alton Station, Booking Hall *(SW Trains)*

DISTRICT COUNCIL
NORTH OXFORDSHIRE

For more information on Toilet
Facilities and Access at all Local
Attractions why not check our website
www.cherwell-gov.uk

---

 the disability rights people

Get Motoring

Your guide to everything the disabled motorist
needs to know about finding, financing and
maintaining a car.

Available from Radar's online shop
www.radar-shop.org.uk

Bordon	Camp Road/High Street A325
	The Forest Shopping Centre *(Private)*
Grayshott	Headley Road Car Park
Horndean	Blendworth Lane Car Park
Liphook	Parish Council Office, Midhurst Rd *(Parish Council)*
Liss	Lower Mead Shops *(Private)*
Petersfield	Central Car Park
	St Peters Road
	Ramswalk (2) *(Private)*
	Petersfield Station, Platform 2 *(SW Trains)*
	'Red Lion', College Street *(JDW)*
Selborne	Car Park, behind Selborne Arms

Eastleigh

Bishopstoke	Bishopstoke Road, Playing Fields
Botley	Mortimer Road Car Park *(Parish Council)*
Chandlers Ford	Winchester Road, The Precinct
	Chandlers Ford Station, Booking Hall *(SW Trains)*
Eastleigh	Bus Station Concourse
	Eastleigh Station, Booking Hall *(SW Trains)*
	'Nandos', Swan Centre *(Nandos)*
	'Wagon Works', Southampton Road *(JDW)*
	AMF Bowl, Swan Centre *(AMF)*
Hamble	Foreshore Car Park
Hedge End	Lower Northam Road *(Town Council)*
Netley	Abbey Hall, Victoria Road
	Royal Victoria Country Park *(Hants CC)*
Southampton Airport	Southampton Airport Station *(SW Trains)*
West End	Itchen Valley Country Park
	Chapel Road *(Parish Council)*

Fareham

Fareham	Trinity Street
	Fareham Shopping Centre, by Shopmobility *(Private)*
	Fareham Shopping Centre, Thackery Mall *(Private)*
	Fareham Station, Booking Hall *(SW Trains)*

	'Crown Inn', West Street *(JDW)*
	'Lord Arthur Lee', West Street *(JDW)*
Hill Head	Cliff Road
	Meon Shore
	Salterns Lane Car Park
Locksheath	Lockswood Centre
Park Gate	Middle Road, by shops
Portchester	Castle Street Car Park, by shops
	Waterside Lane, by Castle
Sarisbury	Holly Hill Woodland Park
Stubbington	Monks Hill
	Stubbington Green
Titchfield	Barry's Meadow, Southampton Hill
Warsash	Passage Lane

Gosport

Gosport	Falkland Gardens
	Forton Recreation Ground [Temp. closed]
	Jamaica Place
	Nobes Avenue [Temp. closed]
	Ordnance Road
	'The Star', High Street *(JDW)*
Lee-on-Solent	Marine Parade Central, Car Park
	Marine Parade East
	Marine Parade West
Stokes Bay	Central
	Gilkicker
	No. 2 Battery

Hart

Eversley Cross	'Frog & Wicket' *(Private)*
Fleet	Church Road Car Park
	Hart Shopping Centre *(Private)*
	Fleet Station, Platform 2 *(SW Trains)*
	'Prince Arthur', Fleet Road *(JDW)*
Hartley Wintney	Car Park, off High Street

| Hook | Car Park, London Road A30 |
| Odiham | 'Waterwitch', Colthill *(Private)* |

Havant

Bedhampton	Bidbury Mead Recreation Ground
Cowplain	Mission Lane Car Park
	Recreation Ground, Padnell Avenue
Emsworth	Recreation Ground, Horndean Road
	South Street Car Park
Havant	Civic Offices
	Havant Park, Havant Parade
	Staunton Country Park *(Hants CC)*
	Meridian Centre, nr. Library *(Private)*
	Havant Bus Station, Elm Lane *(Private)*
	Havant Station, Platform 1 *(SW Trains)*
	'Parchment Makers', Park Rd North *(JDW)*
	AMF Bowling, Havant Retail Park *(AMF)*
Hayling Island	Bosmere Road (Summer only)
	Central Beachlands
	Chichester Avenue
	Eastoke Corner
	Elm Grove
	Ferry Point
	Nab Tower Car Park
	Station Road
	West Beachlands Car Park

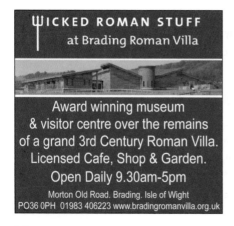
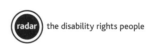 the disability rights people

Get Mobile

Radar's independent guide to help you purchase
a mobility scooter or powered wheelchair.

Available from Radar's online shop
www.radar-shop.org.uk

Langstone	Ship Inn
Leigh Park	Greywell Car Park
Purbrook	Purbrook Heath Recreation Ground
Warblington	Warblington Cemetery (Cemetery hrs)
Waterlooville	Swiss Road
	Waterlooville Cemetery (Cemetery hrs)
	'Woodpecker', London Road *(Private)*

Isle Of Wight

Bembridge	Harold Lewis Day Centre, High Street
	Whitecliff Bay Holiday Park (2) *(Private)*
Binstead	Recreation Ground, Binstead Hill
Brighstone	Warnes Lane Car Park
Carisbrooke	High Street Car Park (Daytime)
Colwell	Colwell Chine Road Car Park
Compton Bay	Military Road Car Park (April-Oct)
Cowes, East	Albany Road (April-Oct)
	Osbourne Road, by Town Hall
	Car Ferry Terminal *(Red Funnel)*
Cowes, West	Cowes Parade
	Cross Street, off High Street
	Medina Road
	Mornington Road (April-Oct)
	Park Road Car Park
	Recreation Ground, Park Road (Apr-Oct)
	Passenger Ferry Terminal *(Red Funnel)*
Freshwater	Moa Place (Daytime)
Godshill	Car Park, High Street
Gurnard	Shore Road
Lake	New Road/High Street (Daytime)
Newport	Church Litten, South Street Car Park
	Post Office Lane
	'William Coppin', Coppins Bridge *(JDW)*
CP	Riverside Centre, The Quay *(Private)*
Ryde	Appley Park, Garden Walk

	Eastern Esplanade (April-Oct) Puckpool Park (Daytime) St Johns Road Town Hall, Lind Street Western Esplanade, The Pier 'S Fowler & Co', Union Street *(JDW)*
St Helens	The Duver (May-September) St Helens Green
Sandown	Battery Gardens (Apr-October) Eastern Gardens (Daytime) Pier Street (M+F) (Daytime) St John's Road Car Park (Daytime) Southland Caravan Club Site *(Caravan Club)*
Seaview	Ropewalk *(Private)*
Shanklin	The Esplanade (Daytime) Falcon Cross Road (M+F) Lake Cliff Gardens, Skew Bridge (Apr-Oct) Rylstone Gardens, Popham Road Tower Cottage Gardens (Daytime) Shanklin Station, Platform *(Island Line)*
Ventnor	Botanic Gardens, Visitor Centre (Centre hrs) Eastern Esplanade (M+F) (Daytime) Marlborough Road (M+F) (Daytime) Pound Lane
Wootton	Car Park, off Brannon Way (Daytime)
Yarmouth	Bridge Road High Street, opp. Common (April-Oct)
Yaverland	Culver Parade Car Park (Daytime)

Milton Keynes

Bletchley	Albert Street *(Neighbourhood Council)* George Street *(Neighbourhood Council)* Bletchley Station, Concourse *(London Midland)*
Caldecotte	'Caldecotte Arms', Bletchern Way *(Private)*
Milton Keynes Central **CP**	the centre:mk *(Private)* Milton Keynes Station, Platforms 3/4 *(London Midland)* 'City Limits', Xscape Village *(Private)* 'Ha! Ha! Bar', Midsummer Boulevard *(Private)*

'Lloyds Bar', Theatre Quarter *(JDW)*
'Nandos', Queens Court, The Centre *(Nandos)*
'Nandos', The Hub *(Nandos)*
'Nandos' Xscape *(Nandos)*
'Moon Under Water', Avebury Boulevard *(JDW)*
'Rat & Parrot', Theatre Quarter *(Private)*
'Secklow Hundred', Midsummer Boulevard *(JDW)*
'Wetherspoons', Bouverie Square *(JDW)*
Cineworld Cinema, Xscape *(Private)*

Newport Pagnell	Market Hill *(Town Council)*
Olney	Market Square *(Town Council)*
Stoney Stratford	Silver Street *(Neighbourhood Council)*
Wolverton	Wolverton Station *(London Midland)*
Wroughton-on-the-Green	'Ye Old Swan', Newport Road *(Private)*

New Forest District Council

Barton-on-Sea	Barton Court Avenue/Marine Drive
Beaulieu	Car Park, Palace Lane
Blackfield	Lepe Country Park *(Hants CC)*
Bransgore	Betsy Lane Car Park

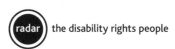 the disability rights people

Doing IT Differently

Part of our 'Doing Life Differently'
series, this toolkit provides
information to help everyone take
advantage of IT.

Available from Radar's online shop
www.radar-shop.org.uk

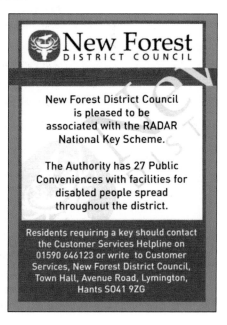

New Forest District Council
is pleased to be
associated with the RADAR
National Key Scheme.

The Authority has 27 Public
Conveniences with facilities for
disabled people spread
throughout the district.

Residents requiring a key should contact
the Customer Services Helpline on
01590 646123 or write to Customer
Services, New Forest District Council,
Town Hall, Avenue Road, Lymington,
Hants SO41 9ZG

	New Forest Caravan Club Site *(Caravan Club)*
Brockenhurst	Fibbards Road Car Park
	Brockenhurst Station, Platform 1 *(SW Trains)*
	Black Knowl Caravan Club Site *(Caravan Club)*
Burley	Chapel Lane Car Park
Calshot	Calshot Spit
Fawley	Car Park
Fordingbridge	Roundhill Car Park
	Sandy Balls Holiday Park *(Private)*
Hythe	Hythe Pier
Keyhaven	Car Park
Lymington	Bath Road Car Park
	New Street
	Powlett Road, M&S Car Park
	Quay Road
Lyndhurst	Car Park, High Street (2)
Milford-on-Sea	Hordle Cliff Car Park
	Hurst Road, Car Park
	Sea Road, Car Park
New Milton	Recreation Ground, Old Milton Road
	Station Road, Car Park
Ringwood	Ringwood Furlong Car Park
Totton	Cemetery Car Park, Eling Hill
	Eling Recreation Ground, Bartram Road
	Library Road
	Winsor Road

Oxford

Oxford	Bury Knowle Park, Headington
	Cowley Road
	Cutteslowe Park
	Diamond Place, Summertown
	Gloucester Green Bus Station
	Market Street
	Oxpens Coach Park
	St Clements
	South Parade, Summertown

Speedwell Street
Westgate Car Park, Level 4
Oxford Station, Concourse *(Gt Western)*
Botanic Garden, Rose Lane *(Private)*
Debenhams Store, Magdalen St *(Debenhams)*
'Four Candles', George Street *(JDW)*
'Jongleurs', Hythe Bridge Road *(Private)*
'Nandos', Cowley Road *(Nandos)*
'Swan & Castle', Castle Street *(JDW)*
'The Victoria', 90 Walton Street *(Private)*
'William Morris', Cowley *(JDW)*
Student Union, Headington Campus *(Oxford Brookes Univ.)*
CP Shopmobility Unit, Westgate Car Park *(Centre hrs)*

Portsmouth

Cosham	Wootton Street 'The First Post', High Street *(JDW)*
Fratton	Clarkes Road (7.00-16.30) Fratton Station, Booking Hall *(SW Trains)* Asda Store, Fratton *(Asda)*
Hilsea	Hilsea Lido
North End	Derby Road 'Sir John Baker', London Road *(JDW)*
Old Portsmouth	Point Battery White Hart Road
Paulsgrove	Marsden Road
Portsmouth	Bransbury Park (7.00-19.00) Buckland Park College Park Guildhall Square (8.00-17.00) The Hard Interchange Milton Park (7.00-17.00) Paradise Street (7.00-19.00) Tangier Road (7.00-19.00) Morrisons Store, Anchorage Road *(Morrison)* Portsmouth & Southsea Station, Concourse *(SW Trains)* Portsmouth Harbour Station, Concourse *(SW Trains)* 'Bar 38', Gun Wharf Quays *(Private)* 'Ha! Ha! Bar', Gun Wharf Quays *(Private)*

'Isambard Kingdom Brunel', Guildhall Walk *(JDW)*
'John Jacques', Fratton Road *(JDW)*
'Jongleurs', Gun Wharf Quays *(Private)*
'Lloyds Bar', The Boardwalk *(JDW)*
'Nandos', Gunwharf Quays *(Nandos)*
'Trafalgar', Edinburgh Road *(JDW)*
'Walkabout', Guildhall Walk *(Private)*
'White Swan', Guildhall Walk *(JDW)*
'Yates's Bar', High Street *(Yates)*
Portsmouth BowlPlex, Gun Wharf Quays *(BowlPlex)*
King Henry Building *(Univ of Portsmouth)*

Southsea Central

Albert Road
Highland Road
Richmond Place
'Lord Palmerston', Palmerston Road *(JDW)*
Langstone Student Village, Bar *(Univ of Portsmouth)*

Southsea Seafront

Canoe Lake
Castlefield
Clarence Pier
D-Day Museum Car Park (April-Sept)
Eastney Esplanade
St Georges Road
South Parade Kiosk (April-September)

Reading

Burghfield M4

Reading East Services, M4 Juncts 11-12 *(Moto)*

Caversham

St Martins Precinct, by Waitrose
'Baron Cadogan', Prospect Street *(JDW)*

Reading

Blagrave Street
Broad Street Mall
Cemetery Junction
Cintra Park Pavilion
Friars Walk
Honey End Lane
Hosier Street, nr. Market
Meadway Precinct
Old Market Place
Oxford Road/Wilson Road
Queens Road Car Park
Thame Side Promenade, Richfield Avenue

Debenhams, The Oracle *(Debenhams)*
Reading Station, Concourse & Platform 4 *(Gt Western)*
'Back of Beyond', Kings Road *(JDW)*
'Bar 12', Station Road *(Private)*
'Bar 38', Oracle Centre *(Private)*
'Cape', Friar Street *(Barracuda)*
'Ha! Ha! Bar', Kings Road *(Private)*
'The Hope Tap', Friar Street *(JDW)*
'Jongleurs', Friar Street *(Private)*
'Monks Retreat', Friar Street *(JDW)*
'Nandos', Riverside, The Oracle *(Nandos)*
'Old Orleans', The Oracle *(Private)*
'Nandos', Friar Street *(Nandos)*
'O'Neill's', Blagrave Street *(M&B)*
'Pavlov's Dog'. St Mary's Butts *(Private)*
'Slug & Lettuce', The Oracle *(Private)*
'Walkabout', Wiston Terrace *(Private)*
'Yates's Bar', Friar Street *(Yates)*
Crescent Road Campus *(Thames Valley Univ)*
Kings Road Campus *(Thames Valley Univ)*
Language Centre, Whiteknights *(Univ of Reading)*
Palmer Building, Whiteknights *(Univ of Reading)*
Sports Park, Whiteknights *(Univ of Reading)*
Students' Union, Whiteknights *(Univ of Reading)*
Urban & Regional Studies, Whiteknights *(Univ of Reading)*

Southcote	Prospect Park, Tilehurst Road
Tilehurst	Kentwood Hill, by the Whitehouse
	'The Bear', Park Lane *(Private)*
Whitley	Northumberland Avenue
	Whitley Street
	Whitley Wood Pavilion, Acre Road

Rushmoor

Aldershot	Aldershot Park, Guildford Road
	Manor Park, High Street/Ash Road
	Wellington Centre *(Private)*
	Aldershot Bus Station *(Private)*
	Aldershot Station, Platform 1 *(SW Trains)*
	'Yates's Bar', Victoria Road *(Yates)*
Farnborough	King George V Playing Fields Pavilion (Daytime)

	Princes Mead *(Private)*
	Farnborough Main Station, Platform 2 *(SW Trains)*
North Camp	High Street

Slough

Langley	East Berkshire College, Langley Centre (4) *(College)*
	Langley Station *(Gt Western)*
Slough	Brunel Bus Station
	The Grove, Slough High Street
	Station Approach
	Observatory Shopping Centre (2) *(Private)*
	Queensmere Centre *(Private)*
	Slough Station, Platform 2 *(Gt Western)*
	'The Moon & Spoon', High Street *(JDW)*
	'Nandos', Queensmere Centre *(Nandos)*
	'Newt & Cucumber', High Street *(Private)*

Southampton

Bitterne	Bitterne Triangle, Cobden Bridge
	Maytree Road, Bitterne Precinct
Lordshill	Gala Bingo, Lordshill Retail Park *(Gala)*
Portswood	Westridge Road
	'Varsity', Portswood Centre *(Barracuda)*
Shirley	'Bright Water Inn', 370 Shirley Road *(JDW)*
	'Malvern Tavern', Winchester Road *(Private)*
CP	Freemantle Community Centre (Centre hrs)

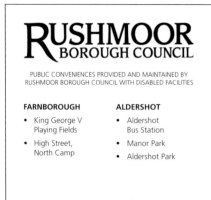

RUSHMOOR BOROUGH COUNCIL

PUBLIC CONVENIENCES PROVIDED AND MAINTAINED BY
RUSHMOOR BOROUGH COUNCIL WITH DISABLED FACILITIES

FARNBOROUGH
- King George V Playing Fields
- High Street, North Camp

ALDERSHOT
- Aldershot Bus Station
- Manor Park
- Aldershot Park

Best wishes from a friend in Oxfordshire

Southampton City Centre	Bargate Street
	East Park Pavilion (Daytime)
	Kingsland Square, St Marys Square
	Mayflower Park
	Poundtree Road
	The Mall Marlands Shopping Centre *(Private)*
CP	West Quay Shopping Centre *(Private)*
	Debenhams Store, Queensway *(Debenhams)*
	Southampton Central Station, Platforms 1 & 4 *(SW Trains)*
	'Admiral Sir Lucius Curtis', Ocean Village *(JDW)*
	'Giddy Bridge' London Road *(JDW)*
	'Jongleurs', Bargate *(Private)*
	'Que Pasa', Above Bar Street *(Marstons)*
	'Standing Order', High Street *(JDW)*
	'Varsity', London Road *(Barracuda)*
	'Yates's Bar', Above Bar Street *(Yates)*
	Mayfield Park
	Weston Shore, Car Park

South Bucks

Beaconsfield	Windsor End, Old Town *(Town Council)*
Burnham	Jennery Lane Car Park *(Parish Council)*
Denham	Wyatts Covert Caravan Site *(Caravan Club)*
Farnham Common	Beaconsfield Road Car Park *(Parish Council)*
	'Royal Oak', Beaconsfield Road *(Private)*
Iver	Iver Garden Centre *(Private)*

South Oxfordshire

Didcot	Orchard Centre (Private)
	Didcot Parkway Station, Platform 2 *(Gt Western)*
Dorchester	Bridge End
Goring	Car Park off Station Road
Henley-on-Thames	Greys Road Car Park
	Kings Road Car Park
	Station Road
	Mill Meadows, Mill Road *(Town Council)*
	'Catherine Wheel', Hart Street *(JDW)*
	Four Oaks Caravan Club Site *(Caravan Club)*

Thame	Market House
	North Street
Wallingford	Cattlemarket Car Park, Wood Street
	Riverside (April-October)
	St Albans Car Park
Watlington	Church Street *(Parish Council)*

Test Valley

Andover	Borden Gate Car Park (Mon-Sat, 8.00-18.00)
	Chantry Centre, by MSCP
	George Yard Car Park (Mon-Sat, 8.00-6.00)
	Andover Station, Platform 1 *(SW Trains)*
	'John Russell Fox', High Street *(JDW)*
Ower	'Vine Inn', Romsey Road *(Private)*
Romsey	Bus Station Car Park, Broadwater Road
Stockbridge	High Street (8.00-18.00) *(Parish Council)*

Vale Of White Horse

Abingdon	Abbey Meadow (April-September, daytime)
	Charter MSCP (Daytime)
Botley	Elms Court, Chapel Way, A35 (Daytime)
Faringdon	Southampton Street Car Park (Daytime)
Wantage	Manor Road Park (Daytime)
	Portway Car Park (Daytime)

West Berkshire

Aldermaston		The Wharf (8.00-18.00 Apr-Sept)
Hungerford		Church Street (8.00-18.00)
Kintbury		Station Road (8.00-18.00)
Lambourn		Community Centre *(Parish Council)*
Newbury	**CP**	Northcroft Leisure Centre (Centre hrs)
		Parkway (8.00-18.00)
		Pembroke Road MSCP (8.00-18.00)
		The Wharf (8.00-18.00)
		Snelsmore Common Country Park (Daytime)
	CP	Kennet Shopping *(Private)*
		Weavers Walk *(Private)*

Newbury Station, Platform *(Gt Western)*
Sainsbury's Store, Hector Way *(Sainsbury)*
'Diamond Tap', Cheap Street *(JDW)*
'Lock Stock & Barrel', Northbrook St *(Fullers)*
Vue Cinema *(Private)*

Pangbourne	River Meadow (April-September, 8.00-18.00)
	Station Road (8.00-18.00)
Thatcham	Broadway (8.00-18.00)
	The Kingsland Centre *(Private)*

West Oxfordshire

Bampton	Town Hall, Market Square
Burford	High Street
	Guildenford Car Park
	Burford Caravan Site *(Caravan Club)*
Carterton	Black Bourton Road, Car Park
Charlbury	Spendlove Centre, Enstone Road (Daytime)
Chipping Norton	New Street, Car Park
	Town Hall, Market Place
Eynsham	Back Lane Car Park
	Oxford Road Playing Field
Witney	Langdale Gate
	The Leys (Daytime)
CP	Windruish Leisure Centre (Centre hrs)

PA Meecham

Are pleased to support Radar

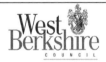

West Berkshire
COUNCIL

All Public Conveniences under our control have
RADAR keys.
They are normally open between 0800 – 1800 daily.

Keys are available from the Market Street,
Council Offices for a small fee.

**For locations or further information
please contact 01635 42400.**
You can also visit our website www.westberks.gov.uk
or West Berkshire Disability Alliance website
www.wbda.org for further information.

Woodstock	Hensington Road Car Park
	Bladon Chains Caravan Site *(Caravan Club)*

Winchester

Bishops Waltham	Central Car Park, Houchin Street
Denmead	Kidmore Lane Car Park
New Alresford	Station Road
Wickham	Station Road
	Rooksbury Park Caravan Club Site *(Caravan Club)*
Winchester	Abbey Gardens, The Broadway
	Chesil Street MSCP
	Discovery Centre, Jewry Street
	Market Lane
	Middle Brook Street
	St Catherines Park & Ride (daytime)
	Tower Street Car Park
	Worthy Lane Coach Station/Car Park
	Brooks Shopping Centre *(Private)*
	Debenhams Store, High Street *(Debenhams)*
	Winchester Station, Platform 2 *(SW Trains)*
	'Bishop on the Bridge', High Street *(Fullers)*
	'Old Gaol House', Jewry Street *(JDW)*
	Morn Hill Caravan Club Site *(Caravan Club)*

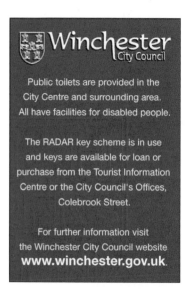

Winchester City Council

Public toilets are provided in the City Centre and surrounding area. All have facilities for disabled people.

The RADAR key scheme is in use and keys are available for loan or purchase from the Tourist Information Centre or the City Council's Offices, Colebrook Street.

For further information visit the Winchester City Council website. **www.winchester.gov.uk**.

Windsor & Maidenhead

Ascot	Station Hill
	Ascot Station, Platform 1 *(SW Trains)*
Cookham	Sutton Road Car Park
Eton	Eton Court Car Park
Hurley	Hurley Riverside Park *(Private)*
Maidenhead	Broadway MSCP (7.30-18.00)
	Providence Place (8.00-18.00)
CP	Magnet Leisure Centre
	Maidenhead Station *(Gt. Western)*
	'Bar 38', Grenfell Island *(Private)*
	'Bear', High Street *(JDW)*
	'Greyhound', Queen Street *(JDW)*
Sunninghill	High Street
Windsor	Coach Park (Daytime)
	River Street Car Park
	Windsor Leisure Centre (Centre hrs)
	East Berkshire College, The Hub *(College)*
	Windsor & Eton Riverside Station, Concourse *(SW Trains)*
	'Ha! Ha! Bar', Windsor Royal Station *(Private)*
	'King & Castle', Thames Street *(JDW)*
	'Nandos', 10 Thames Street *(Nandos)*
	'Windlesora', William Street *(JDW)*

Wokingham

Barkham	'Ye Olde Leathern Bottle', Barkham Rd *(Private)*
Twyford	Twyford Station, Platform *(Gt Western)*
Wokingham	'Gig House', Denmark Street *(JDW)*
	Gala Bingo, Easthampstead Road *(Gala)*

Wycombe

Bourne End	Wakeman Road
Flackwell Heath	Straight Bit
Hambleden	Mill End Car Park
Hazlemere	Beaumont Way
	Park Parade

High Wycombe	Easton Street MSCP
	Pauls Row (Daytime)
	Sainsburys Dovecote MSCP (Daytime)
	Eden Shopping Centre *(Private)*
	Bus Station, Bridge Street *(Private)*
	'The Falcon', Cornmarket *(JDW)*
	'Nandos', Eden Shopping Centre *(Nandos)*
	'William Robert Loosley', Oxford Road *(JDW)*
	AMF Bowl, Eden Centre *(AMF)*
Marlow	Central Car Park, Crown Lane
	Pound Lane (Daytime)
	Marlow Library (Library hrs) *(Bucks CC)*
Princes Risborough	Horns Lane Car Park
West Wycombe	Hill Road

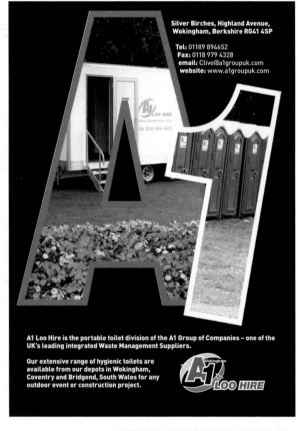

Bath & North East Somerset

Bath City Centre	Charlotte Street Car Park
	Charlotte Street, entrance to Car Park
	Henrietta Park, Henrietta Street
	Parade Gardens, Grand Parade
	Riverside Coach Park, Avon Street
	Royal Victoria Park, Pavilion, Royal Avenue
	Royal Victoria Park, Play Area, Upper Bristol Rd
	Seven Dials, Monmouth Street
	Sydney Gardens, Sydney Place
	Victoria Art Gallery (Gallery hrs)
	Weston High Street, near shops
	Podium Shopping Centre *(Private)*
	Bath Spa Station, Platforms *(Gt Western)*
	'Ha! Ha! Bar', Walcot Street *(Private)*
	'King of Wessex', James Street *(JDW)*
	'Nandos', James Street West *(Nandos)*
	Gala Bingo, Sawclose *(Gala)*
	Newbridge Caravan Park *(Private)*
Bath, Beechen Cliff	Alexandra Park, Shakespeare Avenue
Bath, Combe Down	Bradford Road
Bath, Lambridge	Alice Park, Gloucester Road
	Larkhall Square
Bath, Lansdown	Approach Golf Course, Weston Road

Bristol City Council

fully supports

RADAR

0117 922 2100

www.bristol.gov.uk

Bath & North East Somerset Council

Council Connect

01225 39 40 41

www.bathnes.gov.uk

Bath, Odd Down		Park & Ride Site
Bath, Oldfield Park		Monksdale Road
		Shaftesbury Road
Bath, Twerton		Twerton High Street, by stadium
Batheaston		London Road Car Park *(Parish Council)*
Keynsham		Ashton Way Car Park
		Memorial Park
	CP	Keynsham Leisure Centre (Centre hrs)
Midsomer Norton		Gullock Tyning, by Sports Centre
		The Island, High Street
Paulton		High Street, Red Lion Car Park *(Parish Council)*
Peasedown St John		Greenlands Road, Car Park
Saltford		The Shallows Car Park, picnic area

Bournemouth

Boscombe & Southbourne	Ashley Road Bus Station
	Boscombe Overcliff Gardens
	Fisherman's Walk, Southbourne
	Hengistbury Head, Double Dykes
	Seabourne Road, opp Pokesdown Station
	Southbourne Crossroads
	Tuckton Road, nr Belle Vue Rd
	Wick Lane Car Park, Tuckton
	'Sir Percy Florence Shelley', Christchurch Rd *(JDW)*
	'Yates's Bar', Dean Park Crescent *(Yates)*
Bournemouth	East Overcliffe, opp. Carlton Hotel
	Firbank Road/Charminster Road (2)
	Lower Gardens, Exeter Crescent
	Poole Hill, Ther Triangle
	Richmond Gardens MSCP (Daytime)
	Travel Interchange, by Coach Station
	West Overcliffe, nr West Hill
	Westover Road, by Information Bureau
	Bournemouth Station, Platform 2/3 *(SW Trains)*
	Debenhams Store, The Square *(Debenhams)*
	'Christopher Creeke', Holdenhurst Road *(JDW)*
	'Moon in the Square', Exeter Road *(JDW)*
	'Nandos', Castlepoint *(Nandos)*

'Walkabout', Old Christchurch Rd *(Private)*
Old Fire Station, Landsdowne Campus *(University)*

Kinson Green	Milhams Road (Daytime)
CP	Kinson Hub, Wimborne Rd (Library hrs)

Seafront	Alum Chine, Bournemouth
	Bedford Beach, Southbourne
	Boscombe East
	Boscombe West
	Bournemouth East
	Bournemouth Pier
	Bournemouth West
	Coasters, nr Boscombe Pier
	Durley Chine, Bounemouth

Wallisdown	Old Mulberry Close, Aldi Car Park

Westbourne	Milburn Road Car Park

Winton	Leslie Road
	'Parkstone & Heathlands', Wimborne Rd *(JDW)*
	Gala Bingo, Wimborne Road *(Gala)*

Bristol

Ashton	Ashton Road

Bedminster	Bridgwater Road, Bedminster Down (Daytime)
	East Street
	Victoria Park (Park hrs)
	'Robert Fitzharding', Cannon St. *(JDW)*

Brislington	'White Hart', Brislington Hill *(Private)*

Bristol City Centre	Albion Marina, Hotwells (Daytime)
	Castle Park, Broadweir (Daytime)
	Colston Avenue (8.00-19.00)
	St James Barton (Daytime)
	Wapping Wharf, Redcliff (Daytime)
	The Mall Bristol, Broadmead, (3) *(Private)*
	Bristol Temple Meads Station (3) *(Gt Western)*
	'Bay Horse', Lewind Mead *(Private)*
	'Commercial Rooms', Corn Street *(JDW)*
	'Green House', College Green *(Private)*
	'Jongleurs', Baldwin Street *(Private)*
	'Knights Templar', Temple Quay *(JDW)*

'Nandos', Cabot Circus *(Nandos)*
'Que Pasa', Corn Street *(Marstons)*
'V-Shed', The Waterfront *(JDW)*
'Walkabout, Corn Street *(Private)*
Blue Wharf Aquarium, Anchor Road *(Private)*
Baltic Wharf Caravan Site *(Caravan Club)*

Clifton	Central Museum, Queens Road (Museum hrs)
	'The Berkeley', Queens Road *(JDW)*
	'The Cotham Hill', Cotham Hill *(Private)*
	'Ha! Ha! Bar', Berkeley Square *(Private)*
Fishponds	Fishponds Park (Daytime)
	'Van Dyke Forum', Fishponds Road *(JDW)*
	Gala Bingo, Fishponds Road *(Gala)*
Knowle	Redcatch Park (Park hrs)
Montpellier	St Andrews Park (Park hrs)
Redfield	'St George's Hall', Church Road *(JDW)*
Southmead	Greystoke Avenue (Daytime)
Stoke Bishop	Sea Wall, Durdham Down (Daytime)
	Stoke Road, by Water Tower (Daytime)

Cheltenham

Cheltenham	Ambrose Street/High Street
	Bath Terrace, off Bath Road
	Coronation Square, Car Park
	Cox's Meadow, Old Bath Road
	Imperial Square, by Town Hall

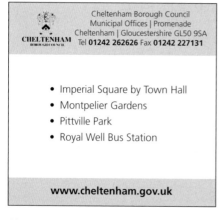

Cheltenham Borough Council
Municipal Offices | Promenade
CHELTENHAM Cheltenham | Gloucestershire GL50 9SA
Tel **01242 262626** Fax **01242 227131**

- Imperial Square by Town Hall
- Montpelier Gardens
- Pittville Park
- Royal Well Bus Station

www.cheltenham.gov.uk

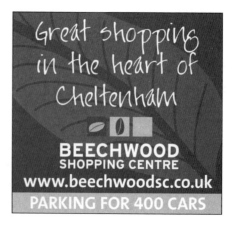

Great shopping in the heart of Cheltenham

BEECHWOOD
SHOPPING CENTRE
www.beechwoodsc.co.uk
PARKING FOR 400 CARS

Montpellier Gardens
Pittville Park
Royal Well Bus Station
Royal Well Road, by Municipal Offices
Beechwood Shopping Centre *(Private)*
Sainsbury's Store, Tewkesbury Rd *(Sainsbury)*
Cheltenham Spa Station *(Gt Western)*
'Bank House', Clarence Street *(JDW)*
'Ha! Ha! Bar', Montpellier Walk *(Private)*
'Moon Under Water', Bath Road *(JDW)*
'Nandos', St Margarets Road *(Nandos)*
'Que Pasa', Clarence St *(Marstons)*
'Yates's Bar', Crescent Terrace *(Yates)*

Christchurch

Christchurch	Bridge Street
	Christchurch Quay (8.00-19.20 or dusk)
	Kings Arms Bowls Pavilion (8.00-18.40 or dusk)
	Saxon Square, off High Street (8.00-18.00)
Friars Cliffe	Promenade, by Beach Café
Highcliffe	Highcliffe Cliffe Top. Cliffhanger (Café hrs)
	Recreation Ground, Wharncliffe Rd (8.00-20.20 or dusk)
	Sea Corner, Waterford Road
Mudeford	Quay Head
	Recreation Ground, Ledbury Road (8.00-21.00 or dusk)
Mudeford Sandbank	Toilet Block 3, nr Ferry Pontoon
	Toilet Block 5, nr Black House (March-October)
Purewell	Purewell Cross Roads

Cotswold

Bibury	London Road (Daytime)
Bourton-on-the-Water	Church Rooms (Daytime)
	Rissington Road Car Park (Daytime)
Chipping Campden	Sheep Street (Daytime)
Cirencester	Brewery Car Park (Daytime)
	Forum Car Park (Daytime)
	London Road (Daytime)
	Lorry Park (Daytime)

	Abbey Grounds (April-Oct) *(Town Council)*
	Cirencester Park Caravan Club Site *(Caravan Club)*
Fairford	High Street (Daytime)
Lechlade	Burford Road (Daytime)
Moreton-in-Marsh	High Street (Daytime)
	Moreton-in-Marsh Caravan Club Site *(Caravan Club)*
Northleach	Market Place (Daytime)
Stow-on-the-Wold	Market Square (Daytime)
	Maugersbury Road Car Park (8.00-21.00)
Tetbury	Chipping Street (Daytime)
	West Street (Daytime)

East Dorset

Ashley Heath	**CP**	Moors Valley Country Park
Corfe Mullen		Towers Way
Ferndown		Pennys Walk
		'The Night Jar', Victoria Road *(JDW)*
Verwood		Ferret Green
West Moors		Park Way
West Parley		Christchurch Road
Wimborne Minster		Cook Row
		Hanham Road, South Car Park

Forest Of Dean

Broomsgreen	Memorial Hall *(Hall Committee)*
Cinderford	Heywood Road Car Park
Coleford	Railway Drive Car Park
Lydbrook	New Road
Lydney	Newerne Street Car Park
Mile End	Mile End Cemetery
Mitcheldean	High Street Car Park
Newent	Lewell Street Car Park, High Street
Newnham-on-Severn	Riverside Car Park
Woolaston	Peters Cross Picnic Area

Gloucester

Gloucester	Berkeley Street
	Gloucester Bus Station
	Gloucester Park (Park hrs)
	Kings Square
	Westgate Car Park
	The Mall Gloucester, East Gate *(Private)*
	Debenhams Store, Kings Sq *(Debenhams)*
	'Nandos', Gloucester Quays Outlet *(Nandos)*
	'The Regal', Kings Square *(JDW)*
	'Sloans', Brunswick Road *(Private)*
	'Varsity', Northgate Street *(Barracuda)*
	'Water Poet', Eastgate Street *(JDW)*
	Gala Bingo, Peel Centre *(Gala)*
Kingsholm	Javelin Park & Ride *(County Council)*
Matson	Robinswood Country Park
Quedgeley	Waterwells Park & Ride *(County Council)*

Mendip

Frome	Market Yard Car Park, Justice Lane
	Merchants Barton *(Town Council)*
	Victoria Park, Weymouth Rd *(Town Council)*
	Frome Station, Platform *(Gt Western)*
Glastonbury	St John's Car Park
	Magdalene Street *(Town Council)*
Shepton Mallet	Commercial Road Car Park
	Collett Park, Park Road *(Town Council)*
Street	Southside Car Park
	Clarks Village (2) *(Private)*
	'The Lantokay', High Street *(JDW)*
Wells	Union Street Car Park
	Princes Road Car Park *(Town Council)*
	Recreation Ground, Silver St *(Town Council)*
	'Kings Head', High Street *(Private)*

North Dorset

Blandford Forum	Marsh & Ham Car Park *(Town Council)*
	Corn Exchange (Centre hrs) *(Town Council)*
Gillingham	High Street Car Park *(Town Council)*
Shaftesbury	Bell Street Car Park *(Town Council)*
Stalbridge	Station Road Car Park *(Town Council)*
Sturminster Newton	Station Road Car Park *(Town Council)*

North Somerset

Clevedon	Chalet Conveniences, Elton Road
	Station Road
	'Crab Apple Inn', Southern Way *(Private)*
Portishead	Lake Grounds, Esplanade Rd (8.00-20.00)
	Wyndham Way Car Park
Uphill	Links Road
Weston-super-Mare	Boulevard, by Library (8.00-19.45)
	Grove Park Car Park (8.00-18.00)
	Locking Road Car Park (8.00-20.00)
	Seafront, opp. Atlantic Hotel (Summer)
	Seafront, opp. Oxford Street
	Seafront, opp. Richmond St (Summer)
	Marine Parade, Sanatorium
	Rozel Seafront (8.00-20.00)
	Sand Bay Bus Terminal
	Weston-super-Mare Station *(Gt Western)*
	'Dragon Inn', Meadow Street *(JDW)*
	'Yates's Bar', Regent Street *(Yates)*
	Country View Caravan Park *(Private)*
Winscombe	Woodborough Road
Worle	The Maltings, High Street

Poole

Branksome	Branksome Chine, Beach Car Park
	Branksome Dene Chine
	Branksome Recreation Ground
	Poole Road
Broadstone	Macaulay Road

Canford Heath	The Pilot Car Park. Adastral Road
	Haymoor Bottom Shopping Centre *(Private)*
Hamworthy	Ashmore Avenue, Hamworthy Park
	Blandford Road, by Co-op
	Lake Pier, Lake Drive (8.00-18.00, longer in Summer)
Holton Heath	Sandford Holiday Park *(Private)*
Parkstone	Alexandra Park Recreation Ground
	Jubilee Road
	Viewpoint, Constitution Hill
Poole	Chapel Lane
	Haven Ferry, Panorama Road
	Kingland Road Bus Station
	Newfoundland Drive, Baiter Park
	Poole Park, Central Park Café
	Poole Park, West Gate (8.00-18.00)
	Whitecliff Recreation Ground
	Poole Station, Booking Hall *(SW Trains)*
	'Lord Wimborne', Lagland Street *(JDW)*
	'Nandos', Tower Park *(Nandos)*
	'Yates's Bar', High Street *(Yates)*
	BowlPlex, Tower Park *(BowlPlex)*
The Quay	Quay Visitors Centre
	Watch Station, nr Lifting Bridge
	Dolphin Quays *(Private)*
	'The Quay', The Quay *(JDW)*

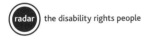
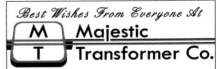

Sandbanks	Banks Road, Sandbanks Pavilion
	Shore Road, Beach Pavilion
Upton Country Park	Upton Heritage Centre (8.00-18.00, longer in Summer)
	Upton Park Car Park (8.00-18.00, longer in Summer)

Purbeck

Corfe Castle	West Street
	Castle Ticket Office *(National Trust)*
Norden	Park & Ride Car Park *(Swanage Rlwy)*
Studland	Beach Road
	Knoll Car Park *(National Trust)*
	Middle Beach *(National Trust)*
	Shell Bay *(National Trust)*
Swanage	Burlington Chine *(Town Council)*
	Heritage Centre (Daytime) *(Town Council)*
	Herston *(Town Council)*
	Shore Road *(Town Council)*
	Haycraft Caravan Club Site *(Caravan Club)*
Wareham	Howards Lane
	Hunters Moon Caravan Club Site *(Caravan Club)*

Sedgemoor

Axbridge	Moorland Street (Daytime)
Berrow	Coast Road (Daytime)
	Hurn Lane Caravan Club Site *(Caravan Club)*
Brean	South Road (Daytime)
	Brean Leisure Park *(Private)*
Bridgwater	Blake Gardens (Mon-Sat, daytime)
	Coach Station, East Quay (Daytime)
	Penel Orlieu
	Taunton Road (Daytime)
	Angel Place Shopping Centre *(Private)*
	'Carnival Inn', St Mary Street *(JDW)*
Bridgwater M5	Bridgwater Services, J24 M5 *(Moto)*
Burnham-on-Sea	Apex Park (Daytime)
	Crosses Penn, Manor Gardens (Daytime)
	Oxford Street Car Park (Daytime)

	South Esplanade, Information Centre (Daytime)
	'The Railway', College Street *(Private)*
	'Reeds Arms', Pier Street *(JDW)*
Cheddar	Cliff Street Car Park (Daytime)
	Dagshole (Daytime)
	Station Road, by School (Daytime)
	Cheddar Caravan Club Site *(Caravan Club)*
Highbridge	Bank Street Car Park (Daytime)
Nether Stowey	Castle Street, Library Car Park *(Parish Council)*
North Petherton	Fore Street, A38 (Daytime)

South Gloucestershire

Alveston	'Ship Inn', Thornbury Road *(Private)*
Aust M48	Severn View Services, J1 M48 *(Moto)*
Charfield	Memorial Hall
Chipping Sodbury	Wickwar Road, Car Park
Cribbs Causeway	'Nandos', Unit 208 Cribbs Causeway *(Nandos)*
Downend	Westerleigh Road
Filton	Church Road
Hanham	Conham River Park
	Laburnham Road, Car Park
	'Nandos', Aspect Leisure Park *(Nandos)*
Kingswood	Kingswood Park, High Street
	Moravian Road (M+F)

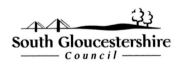

South Gloucestershire
—— *Council* ——

For details of public toilets
in South Gloucestershire
contact

01454 868 000

or visit www.southglos.gov.uk

**Best wishes to
Radar**

	Kingschase Shopping Centre *(Private)*
	'Kingswood Colliers', Regent Street *(JDW)*
Mangotsfield	St James Street Car Park (M+F)
Severn Beach	Beach Road
Staple Hill	Page Park
	Page Road (M+F) (7.30-19.00)
	'Staple Hill Oak', High Street *(JDW)*
Stoke Gifford	Bristol Parkway Station (2) *(Gt Western)*
Thornbury	St Marys Shopping Centre *(Private)*
	'White Lion', High Street *(Private)*
Warmley	Station Yard, High Street
Wick	Golden Valley Shopping Centre *(Private)*
Winterbourne	Flaxpits Lane
Yate	Yate Shopping Centre *(Private)*

South Somerset

Bruton	Grove Alley (Daytime)
Castle Cary	Millbrook Gardens Car Park (Daytime)
	Castle Cary Station *(Gt Western)*
Chard	Bath Street (Daytime)
	Boden Street (Daytime)
	'The Cerdic', Fore Street *(JDW)*
	Five Acres Caravan Club Site *(Caravan Club)*
Crewkerne	South Street
Ilchester	Limington Road/Free Street
Ilminster	Shudrick Lane, nr Tesco (Daytime)
Langport	Whatley Car Park (7.00-19.00) *(Parish Council)*
Martock	Market House, Church Street *(Parish Council)*
Milborne Port	London Road
Somerton	West Street Car Park *(Town Council)*
South Petherton	Prigg Lane (Daytime)
Stoke-sub-Hamdon	Ham Hill (7.00-16.30, later in Summer)
Wincanton	Memorial Hall Car Park (7.00-19.00)
	Carrington Way *(Town Council)*

Churchfields *(Town Council)*
Wincanton Racecourse Caravan Site *(Caravan Club)*

Yeovil
Bus Station, Earle Street (7.00-19.00)
Petters Way Car Park (7.00-19.00)
Recreation Ground, Mudford Road (7.00-19.00)
Peter Street *(Town Council)*
Quedam Centre (Mon-Sat daytime) *(Private)*
'William Dampier', Middle Street *(JDW)*

Stroud

Berkeley	Marybrook Street
Cainscross	Car Park, Westward Rd (Daytime)
Dursley	Castle Street Car Park (Daytime) May Lane Car Park (Daytime)
Kingswood	Rectory Road *(Parish Council)*
Minchinhampton	Bell Lane
Nailsworth	Old Market Bus Station
Painswick	Stamages Lane Car Park St Mary's Street *(Town Council)*
Stonehouse	High Street Car Park
Stroud	Bedford Street Brunel Mall MSCP, London Road (Daytime) Stratford Park, Stratford Road 'The Lord John', Russell Street *(JDW)* 'Old Nelson', Stratford Road *(Private)*
Wotton-under-Edge	Rope Walk (Daytime)

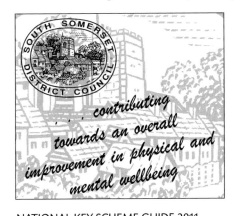

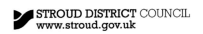
STROUD DISTRICT COUNCIL
www.stroud.gov.uk

For more information on accessibility
to our 12 public conveniences
please visit

www.stroud.gov.uk/docs/environment/
toilets.asp

or call 01453 754549

Swindon

Covingham		Dorcan Way (Mon-Sat, 8.00-16.00)
	CP	Dorcan Recreation Centre (Centre hrs)
Gorse Hill		Chapel Street (Mon-Sat, 8.00-16.00)
Highworth		Brewery Street (Mon-Sat, 8.00-16.00)
		Highworth Recreation Centre (Centre hrs)
Lechlade		Riverside Park (Mon-Sat, daytime)
Middleleaze	CP	Saltway Centre (Centre hrs)
Swindon Town Centre		Brunel Centre, Market Place (Mon-Sat, 9.00-17.30)
		Bus Station, New Bridge Street (Daytime)
	CP	Oasis Leisure Centre (Centre hrs)
		Town Arts Centre, Regent Circus (Centre hrs)
		Town Gardens, Westlecot Street (Park hrs)
		Victoria Road, Old Town (Mon-Sat, 8.00-16.00)
		The Brunel Centre, 1st Floor *(Private)*
		Debenhams Store, The Parade *(Debenhams)*
		House of Fraser Store, Brunel Centre *(Private)*
		Sainsbury's Store, Bridgemead *(Sainsbury)*
		Swindon Station, Platform 1 *(Gt Western)*
		'Bell Hotel', Club Bar *(Private)*
		'Dockle Farmhouse', Bridge End Rd *(JDW)*
		'Groves Company Inn', Fleet Street *(JDW)*
		'The Savoy', Regent Street *(JDW)*
		'Sir Daniel Arms', Fleet Street *(JDW)*
		'Yates's Bar', Bridge Street *(Yates)*
		Gala Bingo, Greenbridge Retail Park *(Gala)*
South Swindon		Barbury Castle Park (Park hrs)
		Coate Water Country Park (Park hrs)
West Swindon		Link Centre (2) (Centre hrs)
		Lydiard Park, Visitor Centre (Park hrs)
		West Swindon Shopping Centre (Mon-Sat, 8.00-16.00)
Wroughton		Wharf Road (Mon-Sat, 8.00-16.00)

Taunton Deane

Bishops Lydeard		Mount Street (8.00-20.00)
		Bishops Lydeard Station *(W Somerset Rly)*
Taunton		Canon Street Car Park (Daytime)

NATIONAL KEY SCHEME GUIDE 2011

Castle Green (M only)
Castle Walk (F only) (Mon-Sat, daytime)
French Weir Recreation Area (Daytime)
High Street MSCP (Daytime)
Paul Street
Station Road, Flook House (Daytime)
Taunton Bus Station (Daytime)
Victoria Park (Daytime)
Vivary Park (Park hrs)
Wilton Lands, nr. Golf Club (Daytime)
Debenhams Store, North St *(Debenhams)*
Sainsbury's Store, Heron Gate *(Sainsbury)*
Taunton Station, Platforms 2 & 5 *(Gt Western)*
'Coal Orchard', Bridge Street *(JDW)*
'Perkin Warbeck', East Street *(JDW)*

Wellington	Longforth Road (Daytime)
	North Street Car Park (Daytime)
	Rockwell Green, Oaken Ground
	Wellington Park (Park hrs)
Wiveliscombe	North Street

Tewkesbury

Alderton	Village Hall (Hall hrs) *(Private)*
Churchdown	Parish Council Offices, Parton Road *(Parish Council)*
Tewkesbury	Bishop Walk, High Street (Town Council)
	Tewkesbury Abbey Caravan Club Site *(Caravan Club)*
Twigworth	'Twigworth', Tewkesbury Road *(Private)*
Winchcombe	Back Lane Car Park *(Parish Council)*

West Dorset

Abbotsbury	Beach *(Private)*
Beaminster	Fleet Street
Bridport	East Street Car Park
	Town Hall
	West Street Car Park
	Eype Picnic Area *(SW Highways)*
	'The Greyhound', East Street *(JDW)*
CP	Bridport Leisure Centre *(Private)*

Buckland Newton	Village Hall *(Parish Council)*
Burton Bradstock	Common Lane Hive Beach *(National Trust)*
Cerne Abbas	Long Street
Charmouth	Foreshore Lower Sea Lane Car Park
Chideock	Sea Hill Lane, Seatown
Dorchester	Maumbury Road, Car Park Old Market Top o' Town Car Park Trinity Street Car Park Waitrose Car Park Kingston Pond, A35 *(SW Highways)* Dorchester South Station, Booking Hall *(SW Trains)* Antelope Walk *(Private)* 'Royal Oak', High West Street *(JDW)* Crossways Caravan Club Site *(Caravan Club)*
Lyme Regis	Broad Street Charmouth Road (Summer) Holmbush Monmouth Beach Marine Parade (Summer) *(Town Council)* Woodmead Car Park *(Town Council)*
Sherborne	Culverhayes Car Park Digby Road Old Market Yard Car Park
West Bay	East Beach Fisherman's Green West Bay Road, Visitors Centre Groves Garden Centre *(Private)*
West Bexington	Beach Car Park

West Somerset

Blue Anchor	Seafront, Central
Dulverton	Lion Stables Car Park Exmoor House Caravan Club Site *(Caravan Club)*
Dunster	Dunster Steep Car Park

Exebridge	Lakeside Caravan Club Site *(Caravan Club)*
Kilve	Kilve Beach Car Park
Minehead	Blenheim Gardens
	Summerland Car Park
	Warren Road, Arcade
	Warren Road, opp. Butlins
	Minehead Station *(W Somerset Rly)*
	'Duke of Wellington', Wellington Square *(JDW)*
	Minehead Caravan Club Site *(Caravan Club)*
Porlock	Central Car Park
	Doverhay Car Park
Tarr Steps	Tarr Steps Car Park *(Exmoor NP)*
Watchet	Harbour Road
	Market Street Car Park
Wheddon Cross	Rest & Be Thankful Car Park *(Parish Council)*
Williton	Car Park, Killick Way

Weymouth & Portland

Portland	Easton Gardens
	Ferrybridge Car Park
	Portland Bill Car Park
	Castletown *(Private)*
Weymouth	Brunswick Terrace, Greenhill
	Cove Street, Hope Square
	The Esplanade
	Lodmoor Car Park, Preston Road
	Nothe Gardens, Barrack Road (Daytime)
	Swannery Car Park, Radipole Park Drive (Daytime)
	Lower St Albans Street MSCP *(Private)*
	Weymouth Station, Booking Hall *(SW Trains)*
	Debenhams Store, New Bond St *(Debenhams)*
	Jubilee Business Park Café *(Private)*
	'Que Pasa', St Thomas St *(Marstons)*
	'The Swan', St Thomas Street *(JDW)*
	'William Henry', Frederick Place *(JDW)*
	'Yates's Bar', St Thomas Street *(Yates)*
	Gala Bingo, Crescent Street *(Gala)*

Wiltshire

Amesbury	Central Car Park
Bradford-on-Avon	St Margaret's Car Park
	Station Car Park
Calne	The Pippin
Castle Combe	The Street
Chippenham	Bath Road Car Park
	Borough Parade
	Monkton Park
	Sainsbury's Store, Bath Road *(Sainsbury)*
	'Bridge House', Borough Parade *(JDW)*
Corsham	Newlands Road (M+F)
Cricklade	off High Street
Devizes	The Green
	West Central Car Park
	'Silk Mercer', St Johns Street *(JDW)*
Downton	The Borough
Kington Langley	A429 Picnic Site
Lacock	Red Lion Car Park *(National Trust)*
Leigh Delamere M4	Leigh Delamere Services E, J17/18 M4 *(Moto)*
	Leigh Delamere Services W, J17/18 M4 *(Moto)*
Marlborough	George Lane
Melksham	Bath Road Car Park
	Church Street Car Park

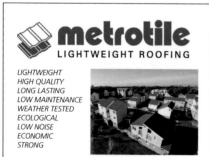

NATIONAL KEY SCHEME GUIDE 2011

	Town Square
Mere	Salisbury Street Car Park
Salisbury	Bemerton Recreation Ground
	Central Car Park
	Churchill Gardens
	Coach Station
	Culver Street
	Guildhall (Guildhall hrs)
	Hudsons Field Campsite (April-October)
	Lush House, Crane Street
	Victoria Park
	Salisbury Cathedral, off Cloisters *(Cathedral)*
	Old George Mall Shopping Precinct *(Private)*
	Debenhams Store, Market Place *(Debenhams)*
	Salisbury Station, Platforms 2 & 4 *(SW Trains)*
	'King's Head', Bridge Street *(JDW)*
	Gala Bingo, Endless Street *(Private)*
	Hillside Caravan Club Site *(Caravan Club)*
Steeple Langford	A36 Picnic Lay-by
Tisbury	Nadder Close
Trowbridge	Trowbridge Park
	'Albany Palace', Park Road *(JDW)*
	'Sir Isaac Pitman', Market Place *(JDW)*
Warminster	Central Car Park
	Warminster Park
	Longleat Caravan Club Site *(Caravan Club)*
Westbury	High Street Car Park
	Warminster Road Car Park
	Westbury Station, Platform 1 *(Gt Western)*
Wilton	Greyhound Lane
Wootton Bassett	Boroughfields Car Park

Cornwall

Bodmin		Lanivet Car Park
		Dennison Road *(Town Council)*
		Fair Park *(Town Council)*
		Priory Park *(Town Council)*
		Bodmin Parkway Station *(Gt Western)*
		'Chapel an Gansblydhen', Fore Street *(JDW)*
Boscastle		Cobweb Car Park
Bude		Crackington Haven
		The Crescent Car Park
		Crooklets Beach Car Park
		Ploughill
		Summerleaze Beach
		Summerleaze Car Park
		Widemouth Bay
		Duckpool, Car Park *(National Trust)*
Callington		New Road
Calstock		The Quay
Camborne		Camborne Park
		Gurneys Lane
		Rosewarne Car Park
Camelford		Enfield Park
Coverack		Car Park (M+F)
Delabole		High Street
Downderry		Main Road
Falmouth	**CP**	Falcare Centre (Centre hrs)
	CP	Ships & Castle Centre (Centre hrs)
		'Packet Station', The Moor *(JDW)*
Gunnislake		by Car Park (M+F) (Daytime)
Gunwalloe		Church Cove (Easter-Sept)
Gwithian		Godrevy *(National Trust)*
Hayle		Foundry Square
		Godrevy Park Caravan Club Site *(Caravan Club)*

Helford		Car Park
Helston		Coinagehall Street
		Trengrouse Way
Kilkhampton		Market Square Car Park
Kingsand		behind Halfway House (F only)
Kynance Cove		Car Park (Easter-Sept) *(National Trust)*
Lanlivery	**CP**	Vitalise Churchtown *(Private)*
Lanner		Playing Field
Launceston		Cattle Market
		Walk House Car Park
Lelant Saltings		Park & Ride (Summer)
Liskeard		Sungirt Car Park
		Westbourne Car Park
		Liskeard Station *(Gt Western)*
Lizard		The Green, Car Park
Looe		Guildhall
		Hannafore
		Millpool
		Seafront
		Looe Caravan Club Site *(Caravan Club)*
Marazion		Station Car Park
Menheniot		East Road *(Parish Council)*
Minions		[No specific information available]
Mullion		Cove (Easter-Sept)
		Village Car Park
Newquay		Newquay Station *(Gt Western)*
		'Sailors Arms', Fore Street *(Private)*
		'Towan Blystra', Cliff Road *(JDW)*
		'Walkabout', The Crescent *(Private)*
Padstow		Council Offices Car Park
		Link Road Car Park
		South Quay
Padstow Coast		Constantine Beach Car Park
		Corys Shelter (F only)
		Harlyn Beach

	Porthcothan Beach
	Trevone Beach
	Treyarnon Beach
Pelynt	Village Hall *(Parish Council)*
Pendeen	Boscaswell (Daytime)
Penzance	Alexandra Gardens (Daytime)
	Jennings Street (Daytime)
	Penalverne, nr. St Johns Hall (Daytime)
	Tourist Information Centre (Daytime)
	Wherrytown, Promenade (Daytime)
	Wharfside Shopping Centre *(Private)*
	Penzance Station *(Gt Western)*
	'Tremenheere', Market Place *(JDW)*
CP	Penzance Childrens Centre
Perranporth	'Green Parrot', St George's Hill *(JDW)*
Poldhu	Beach (Easter-Sept)
Polperro	Fishna Bridge
Polruan	St Saviours
Polzeath	opp. The Beach
	Daymer Beach
	New Polzeath Car Park
Port Isaac	Clifftop Car Park
	Fish Cellars, Roscarrick Hill
Porthallow	Porthallow Beach
Porthcurno	Car Park

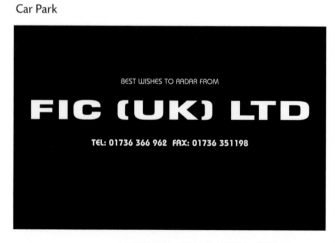

BEST WISHES TO RADAR FROM

FIC (UK) LTD

TEL: 01736 366 962 FAX: 01736 351198

NATIONAL KEY SCHEME GUIDE 2011

Porthleven	Shute Lane
Portreath	Beach Road
Portscatho	Merrose Farm Caravan Club Site *(Caravan Club)*
Poughill	[No specific information available]
Praa Sands	Car Park
Praze-an-Beeble	The Square
Redruth	Fairfield (Events only)
	New Cut Car Park
	Redruth Station, Platform 2 *(Gt Western)*
	Globe Vale Holiday Park *(Private)*
Rejerrah	Monkey Tree Holiday Park *(Private)*
Rose	Treamble Valley Caravan Club Site *(Caravan Club)*
St Austell CP	Priory Road Car Park
	St Austell Station, Platform 1 *(Gt Western)*
	'Rann Wartha', Biddicks Court *(JDW)*
St Ives	Porthmeor Car Park (Daytime)
	Sloop Car Park (May-Sept, daytime)
	Station Car Park (Daytime)
	Trenwith Car/Coach Park (Daytime)
	West Pier (Daytime)
St Just	Lafrowda Close Car Park
St Keverne	The Square
St Merryn	Harlyn Road
St Teath	Car Park, opp White Hart Inn

Globe Vale Holiday Park

Globe Vale is a family run countryside park situated on the North Coast of Cornwall. Facilities include:

* Fully serviced pitches on level hardstanding
* Modern shower/toilet facilites including Disabled shower room
* Bar serving meals – open during peak periods
* Childrens Play Area

Close to local beaches, access to the Coast to Coast Cycle trail. An excellent base to explore attractions including The Eden Project, St Ives and Penzance etc.

For more information contact:
Paul and Louise Owen 01209 891183
www.globevale.co.uk
Email: info@globevale.co.uk

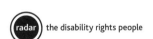 the disability rights people

Doing Work Differently

Part of our 'Doing Life Differently' series, this toolkit explores practical solutions to real questions related to work.

Available from Radar's online shop
www.radar-shop.org.uk

Saltash		Bellevue Car Park
		Longstone Park (M+F) (Daytime)
Sennen		Sennen Cove Car Park (Summer)
Torpoint		Antony Road
		Thanckes Park
		Ferry Queuing Lanes *(Torpoint Ferry)*
Tintagel		Bossinney
		The Castle
		Fore Street, Trevenna Square
		Trerammett
		Visitor Centre
		Trewethett Farm Caravan Club Site *(Caravan Club)*
Trebarwith		Trebarwith Strand
Truro		Truro Station, Platform 2 *(Gt Western)*
		'Barley Sheaf', Old Bridge Street *(Private)*
		'Try Dower', Lemon Quay *(JDW)*
Wadebridge	CP	Camel Trail, Eddystone Road
		Egloshayle Road
		Goldsworthy Way Car Park
		The Platt

East Devon

Axminster	West Street Car Park
Beer	Jubilee Gardens
Branscombe	Beach Car Park
	Village Hall Car Park
Broadclyst	Victory Hall Car Park
Budleigh Salterton	Brook Road Car Park (F only)
	East End, Lime Kiln Seafront
Colyton	Dolphin Street Car Park
Exmouth	Bus/Rail Station (M+F)
	Elizabeth Hall Grounds
	Foxholes Car Park
	Imperial Grounds, opp Car Park
	Lifeboat
	Maer Park
	Magnolia Centre Car Park

	Manor Gardens, by Town Hall
	Phear Park
	Templetown
	'Powder Monkey', The Parade *(JDW)*
Honiton	King Street Car Park
	Lace Walk Car Park
Lympstone	Underhill Car Park
Newton Poppleford	School Lane Car Park
Otterton	The Square
Ottery St Mary	Flexton, Town Centre
	Hind Street Car Park
Seaton	Chine, west of West Walk Esplanade
	Harbour Road Car Park
	Marsh Road, by Town Hall
	West Walk
Sidmouth	Connaught Gardens
	Market Place
	Port Royal
	Triangle
	Long Park, Woolbrook
	Putts Corner Caravan Club Site *(Caravan Club)*

Exeter

Exeter City Centre		Blackboy Road
		King William Street
		Musgrave Row
		Paris Street
		The Quay
	CP	Princesshay Exeter, Catherine St *(Private)*
		Exeter St Davids Station *(Gt Western)*
		'Butlers', Mary Arches Street *(Private)*
		'George's Meeting House', South St *(JDW)*
		'The Imperial', New North Road *(JDW)*
		'Nandos', 32 Princess Hay *(Nandos)*
		'Pitcher & Piano', Queen Street *(Private)*
		'Walkabout', Fore Street *(Private)*
Exeter St Thomas		Cowick Barton Playing Fields
		Cowick Street Railway Arch

	Okehampton Street
	St Thomas Pleasure Ground
	'Sawyers Arms', Cowick Street *(JDW)*
Exwick	Ennerdale Way
Heavitree	Fore Street
	Heavitree Park
Matford	Park & Ride
Polsloe	Hamlin Lane
	'Railwayman', Pinhoe Road *(Private)*
Topsham	Fore Street
	Topsham Quay
Whipton	Pinhoe Road, nr. shops

Isles Of Scilly

| **St Mary's** | Old Weslyan Chapel, Garrison Lane |

Mid Devon

Bampton	Luke Street
Chawleigh	Village Hall (Daytime)
Crediton	Market Street
	Newcombes Meadow
	'General Sir Redvers Buller', High St *(JDW)*
Cullompton	Station Road
Down St Mary	Morchard Road, A377 Picnic Area
Hemyock	Culmbridge Road, by Parish Hall
Sampford Peverell	Recreation Ground
	Tiverton Parkway Station *(Gt Western)*
Tiverton	Lowman Green
	Market Car Park
	Peoples Park
	Phoenix Lane
	Westexe South
	Canal Basin Car Park *(Devon CC)*
	'White Ball Inn', Bridge Street *(JDW)*

North Devon

Blackmoor Gate	Car Park, A399 *(Exmoor NP)*
Barnstaple	Old Cattlemarket Car Park Pannier Market Pilton Park Rock Park North Devon Library & Record Office *(Devon CC)* Green Lanes Shopping Centre *(Private)* Sainsbury's Store, Gratton Way *(Sainsbury)* 'Panniers', Boutport Street *(JDW)* 'Water Gate', The Strand *(JDW)*
Braunton	Caen Street Car Park
Combe Martin	Kiln Car Park
Croyde	Croyde Beach Down End Car Park
Ilfracombe	Bicclescombe Park The Cove The Pier Town Council Offices Wilder Road Car Park
Instow	Marine Drive Car Park Sandy Lane
Mortehoe	Damage Barton Caravan Club Site *(Caravan Club)*
Saunton	Beach Toilets
South Molton	Pannier Market (Daytime)

NORTH DEVON COUNCIL

For more information on
Public Facilities and access to many
attractions why not telephone for
more details before you travel?

Please telephone for all enquiries:

01271 318 501

www.northdevon.gov.uk

For information on Plymouth City
Council public conveniences with
access for the disabled, why not
contact Street Services?

Waste Enquiry Line
01752 668000

Email:
streetservices@plymouth.gov.uk

Visit: www.plymouth.gov.uk

Woolacombe	Willingcott Caravan Club Site *(Caravan Club)*

Plymouth

City Centre		Armada Way, off Ladies (Daytime)
		Central Park, Mayflower Drive
		Civic Centre, Royal Parade (Office hrs)
		Barbican, Quay (Daytime)
		Bretonside Bus Station, off Gents (Daytime)
		Hoe Promenade (Daytime)
		Midland House, Notte Street (Office hrs)
		Phoenix Wharf (Daytime)
		Plymouth Market, Cornwall Street (Market hrs)
		Tinside Lido, The Barbican (Lido hrs)
		Tavistock Road, by Library (Daytime)
		West Hoe (Daytime)
		Devon Housing Aid Centre, Mayflower St *(Shelter)*
		Debenhams Store, Royal Parade *(Debenhams)*
		House of Fraser Store, Royal Parade *(HoF)*
	CP	Drake Circus Shopping Centre *(Private)*
		Plymouth Station, Platform 4 *(Gt Western)*
		'Discovery Café', Eastlake Street *(Private)*
		'Gog & Magog', Southside Street *(JDW)*
		'Ha! Ha! Bar', Princess Street *(Private)*
		'Hogshead', Royal Parade *(Private)*
		'Nandos', Barbican Leisure Park *(Nandos)*
		'The Union Rooms', Union Street *(JDW)*
		'Varsity', Derry's Cross *(Barracuda)*
		'Walkabout', Derry's Cross *(Private)*
		'Watering Hole', Quay Road, Barbican *(Private)*
		Gala Bingo, Derrys Cross *(Gala)*
		Vue Cinema, Barbican Leisure Park *(Private)*
Crown Hill		'KFC', Crown Hill Retail Park *(KFC)*
		'Tamar', Moorshead Road *(Private)*
Devonport		Ferry Approach Lanes *(Torpoint Ferry)*
Estover		Asda Store, Estover Shopping Centre *(Asda)*
Jennycliff		Jennycliff Car Park (Daytime)
Lipson		Freedom Park (Café hrs)
Marsh Mills		Coypool Park & Ride (Daytime)
Mawnamead		Hartley Park

Milehouse	'Britannia Inn', Wolseley Street *(JDW)*
Mount Wise	Mutton Cove (May-September)
Mutley	Mutley Plain 'The Mannamead', Mutley Plain *(JDW)*
Plympton	Ridgeway, Plymco Car Park (Daytime)
Plymstock	Dean Hill (Daytime)
St Budeaux	Wolseley Road
Stoke	Masterman Road (Daytime)
Stonehouse	Cremyll Street (Daytime) Devil's Point (Daytime)
Tamar Bridge	Bridge Car Park, A38 *(Tamar Bridge)*
Turnchapel	Lawrence Road, Mountbatten Car Park (Daytime)

South Hams

Modbury	Broad Park Caravan Club Site *(Caravan Club)*
Stoke Gabriel	Ramslade Caravan Club Site *(Caravan Club)*
Stokenham	Start Bay Caravan Club Site *(Caravan Club)*
Totnes	Totnes Station *(Gt Western)*

Teignbridge

Abbotskserwell	Bottom of Church Path
Ashburton	Kingsbridge Lane Car Park
Bovey Tracey	Station Road

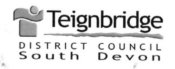

Teignbridge
DISTRICT COUNCIL
South Devon

For more information on toilet
facilities and access, why not
telephone before you travel?

Please telephone for all enquiries:

01626 215 838

Buckfastleigh		Coach Park
Dawlish		Barton Hill
		Boat Cove (Daytime)
		The Lawn, by Tourist Information Centre
		Sandy Lane (Daytime)
		Dawlish Station, Platform 2 *(Gt Western)*
Dawlish Warren		Beach Road Car Park
		Sea Front
Newton Abbot	**CP**	Cricketfield Car Park
		Decoy Country Park, Car Park
		Market Walk
		Newfoundland Way
		Newton Abbot Station, Platform 3 *(Gt Western)*
		'Richard Hopkins', Queen Street *(JDW)*
Shaldon		The Strand
Starcross		The Strand (Summer, daytime)
Teignmouth		Brunswick Street
		Lower Brook Street (Daytime)
		Teignmouth Station, Platform 1 *(Gt Western)*
Widecombe		The Green Car Park

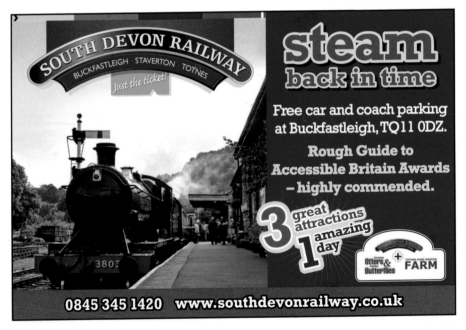

Torbay

Brixham	Bank Lane (Daytime)
	Berry Head
	Brixham Harbour (Daytime)
	Shoalstone Beach (April-October, Daytime)
	'The Vigilance', Bolton Street *(JDW)*
	Hillhead Holiday Park *(Caravan Club)*
Paignton	Broadsands Beach (Daytime)
	Festival Apollo (April-October, Daytime)
	Goodrington Central (Daytime)
	Palace Avenue (8.00-20.00)
	Paignton Central (Daytime)
CP	Paignton Library (Library hrs)
	Parkside/Victoria Square (Daytime)
	Preston North, Marine Drive (Daytime)
	Quaywest Central *(Private)*
	'The Isaac Merritt', Torquay Road *(JDW)*
	'Noahs ArK', Totnes Road *(Private)*
	'Talk of the Town', Torbay Road *(JDW)*
	Gala Bingo, Temperance Street *(Gala)*

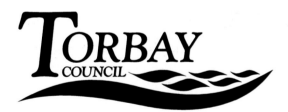

is committed
to being accessible
to all
www.torbay.gov.uk/disability

Torquay	Abbey Meadows (April-October, 9.00-19.00)
	Beacon Quay (Daytime)
	Corbyn Head (April-October, 9.00-19.00)
	Factory Row, off Union Street (Daytime)
	Lymington Road, Coach Station (Daytime)
	Meadfoot Beach (April-October, 9.00-19.00)
	Oddicombe Beach (April-October, 9.00-19.00)
	Old Town Hall, Union Street (Daytime)
	St Marychurch Town Hall, Manor Road (7.00-21.00)
	Seafront Complex (Daytime)
	Vaughan Parade (Daytime)
	Cockington Car Park *(Private)*
	Fleet Walk Shopping Centre *(Private)*
	Torquay Station, Platform 1 *(Gt Western)*
	'Babbacombe Inn', Babbacombe Downs *(Private)*
	'Bar Med', Fleetwalk Centre *(Private)*
	'London Inn', The Strand *(JDW)*
	'Manor Inn', Market Street *(Private)*
	'Shiraz', Vaughan Parade *(Private)*
	Torquay Bowl, Torwood Street *(AMF)*

Torridge

Appledore	Churchfields Car Park (Daytime)
Bideford	Bideford Quay
	Victoria Park (8.00-18.00)
Bradworthy	The Square
Halwill Junction	Playing Field
Holsworthy	North Road
Torrington	The Commons (Daytime)
	South Street (Daytime)
Westward Ho!	Main Putting Green (Daytime)
	Slipway Car Park (Daytime)
Winkleigh	Castle Street

West Devon

Chagford	The Square (Daytime)
Horrabridge	Magpie Car Park (Summer)
Meldon	Meldon Quarry Station *(Dartmoor Rlwy)*

Okehampton	Fairplace, George Street
	Market Street, by Taxi Rank
	Mill Road Car Park
	Okehampton Station *(Dartmoor Rlwy)*
Princetown	Information Centre Car Park
Tavistock	Bedford Car Park, The Wharf
	Guildhall Car Park
	Tavistock Wharf
Yelverton	Roundabout Car Park

Babergh

Chelmondiston	Pin Mill
East Bergholt	Flatford Visitor Centre
	Red Lion Car Park
Lavenham	Cock Inn Car Park
	Prentice Street Car Park
Long Melford	Cordell Road
	The Green
Rodbridge	Rodbridge Picnic Site *(Suffolk CC)*
Sudbury	'Grover & Allen', North Street *(JDW)*

Basildon

Basildon	Basildon Library (Library hrs) *(Essex CC)*
	Eastgate Business Centre (3) *(Private)*
	Eastgate Shopping Centre (3) *(Private)*
	Market Square *(Private)*
	Basildon Station, Booking Hall *(C2C)*
	'Moon on the Square', Market Square *(JDW)*
	'Nandos', Eastgate *(Nandos)*
	'Nandos', Festival Leisure Park *(Nandos)*
	'Towngate', Westgate Park *(Private)*
	Nethermayne Campus *(Thurrock & Basildon College)*
Billericay	Norsey Wood Nature Reseve (Park hrs)
	'Blue Boar', High Street *(JDW)*
	'Red Lion', High Street *(Private)*
Laindon	Shopping Centre (M+F) (Mon-Sat, daytime)
	Laindon Station, Platform 3 *(C2C)*
Pitsea	Watt Tyler Country Park (Park hrs)
	Pitsea Station, Booking Hall *(C2C)*
Wickford	Woodford Road (Mon-Sat, 8.00-16.30)
	Downtowner Youth Centre (Centre hrs) *(Essex CC)*
	The Willows Shopping Centre *(Private)*
	Wickford Station *(NX East Anglia)*
	Royal British Legion Club *(RBL)*

Bedford

Bedford Town Centre	Allhallows Bus Station (M+F) (7.00-18.30)
	Bedford Park East
	Corn Exchange (when open)
	Lurke Street (8.30-17.15)
	Riverside Square (8.15-17.30)
	St Pauls Square (8.00-18.00)
	Debenhams Store, High Street *(Debenhams)*
	Bedford Station, Platform 1 *(Capital Connect)*
	'Bankers Draft', High Street *(JDW)*
	'Nandos', High Street *(Nandos)*
	'Pilgrims Progress', Midland Road *(JDW)*
	'Que Pasa', St Pauls Square *(Marstons)*
East Bedford	Priory Country Park (8.00-18.00)
	Russell Park (8.00-17.00, later in Summer)
Kempston	Addison Howard Park (Park hrs)

Braintree

Braintree	Victoria St. Bus Park (8.00-17.00)
	Braintree Library, Fairfield Rd (Library hrs) *(Essex CC)*
	Braintree Station, Ticket Office *(NX East Anglia)*
	'Baileys Café Bar', High Street *(Private)*
	'Picture Palace', Fairfield Road *(JDW)*
	'Silk Worm', High Street *(Private)*
	CP Charles Leeks House, Coggeshall Road *(Mencap)*
Castle Hedingham	Memorial Lane (8.00-17.00)
Earls Colne	Queens Road Car Park (8.00-17.00)
Finchingfield	Stephen Marshall Avenue (8.00-17.00)
Witham	Lockrams Lane (8.00-17.00)
	Witham Library (Library hrs) *(Essex CC)*
	Witham Station *(NX East Anglia)*
	'Battesford Court', Newland Street *(JDW)*

Breckland

Attleborough	Queens Square, Car Park (Daytime) *(Town Council)*
Dereham	Barwells Court, Market Place *(Town Council)*
	Cowper Road, Car Park (Daytime) *(Town Council)*
Roudham Heath	Rest Area *(Highway Authority)*

Swaffham	The Shambles, Market Place *(Town Council)*
Thetford	Bridge Street Car Park *(Town Council)*
	Cage Lane *(Town Council)*
	Castle Park, Castle Street *(Town Council)*
Watton	St Giles Car Park (Daytime) *(Town Council)*

Brentwood

Brentwood	Brentwood Station
	High Street (7.30-19.30)
	'Nandos', High Street *(Nandos)*
Ingatestone	Market Place (Mon-Sat, 8.00-18.00)
Shenfield	Shenfield Station, Platform 3 *(NX East Anglia)*
West Horndon	West Horndon Station, Ticket Hall *(C2C)*

Broadland

Acle	The Street, by Kings Head
Ranworth	The Staithe, opp. The Maltsters (April-October)
Salhouse	Salhouse Broad Car Park (M+F) (April-Oct)

Limbless Association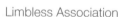

We are a leading UK charity for people with limb-loss, their family, friends and carers. We offer free, friendly and impartial information on all aspects of limb-loss.

Tel. 01277 725186

www.limbless-association.org

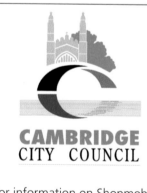

CAMBRIDGE CITY COUNCIL

For information on Shopmobility and public toilets:

Visit our website
www.cambridge.gov.uk
or contact our
customer service centre:
Telephone 01223 458282

| Thorpe St Andrew | River Green, Yarmouth Road (April-Oct) |

Broxbourne

| Broxbourne | Deaconsfield, High Road |
| | Old Mill Meadows Car Park *(Lee Valley RPA)* |

Cheshunt	Grundy Park, Turners Hill (Daytime)
	Pindar Car Park *(Lee Valley RPA)*
	'King James', Turners Hill *(JDW)*

| Hoddesdon | Tower Centre, Amwell Street (Daytime) |

Waltham Cross	High Street, Car Park (Daytime)
	Highbridge Car Park *(Lee Valley RPA)*
	'The Moon & Cross', High Street *(JDW)*

Cambridge

Cambridge	Arbury Court, nr. shops (8.00-19.00)
	Cherry Hinton Hall (Daytime)
	Chesterton Recreation Ground (Daytime)
	Chesterton Road, by Mitcham's Corner (Daytime)
	Coleridge Recreation Ground (April-Oct, daytime)
	Corn Exchange (2) (Centre hrs)
	Drummer Street Bus Station (8.00-20.00)
	Guildhall, Market Square (Office hrs)
	Jesus Green (Daytime)
	Kings Hedges Recreation Ground (April-Oct, daytime)
	Lammas Land, nr Paddling Pool (Daytime)
	Lion Yard Shopping Centre (8.30-20.00)
	Nightingale Recreation Ground (Daytime)
	Park Street MSCP (8.00-20.00)
	Quayside, off Bridge Street (8.00-20.00)
	Romsey Recreation Ground (8.00-18.00)
	Silver Street, by bridge (8.00-19.00)
	Grafton Centre, by Shopmobility *(Private)*
	Grafton Centre, Eden Court *(Private)*
	Debenhams Store, Grafton Centre *(Debenhams)*
	Cambridge Station, Platform 1 *(NX East Anglia)*
	'McDonalds', Rose Crescent *(McDonalds)*
	'Nandos', Cambridge Leisure Park *(Nandos)*
	'Nandos', St Andrews Street *(Nandos)*
	'Rat & Parrot'', Downing Street *(Private)*
	'The Regal', St Andrew's Street *(JDW)*

'The Tivoli', Chesterton Road *(JDW)*
Helmore Building, East Road *(Anglia Ruskin University)*
Mumford Theatre (Theatre hrs) *(Private)*
Cherry Hinton Caravan Club Site *(Caravan Club)*
CP Grand Arcade Car Park *(Shopmobility)*

Castle Point

Benfleet

Richmond Hall
Tarpot Car Park, Rushbottom Lane
Benfleet Station, Platform 1 *(C2C)*

Canvey Island

Knightswick Shopping Centre
Labworth, Western Esplanade
Lubbins Car Park, Eastern Esplanade

Hadleigh

Rectory Road, CarPark

Central Bedfordshire

Biggleswade

Market Square *(Town Council)*
CP Saxon Pool & Leisure Centre *(Private)*

Dunstable

Ashton Square Car Park, off West Street
'Gary Cooper', Grove Park *(JDW)*
'Sugar Loaf', High Street North *(Private)*

Houghton Regis

Bedford Square

Leighton Buzzard

West Street MSCP
Leighton Buzzard Station, Booking Hall *(London Midland)*

Potton

Brook End, nr. Market Square *(Town Council)*

Shefford

Northbridge Street *(Town Council)*

Stotfold

Brook Street Car Park *(Town Council)*

Toddington M1

Toddington Services, J11/12 M1 *(Moto)*

Chelmsford

Boreham

'Grange', Main Road *(Private)*

Chelmsford

Admirals Park, near footbridge (Daytime)
Central Park, by Bowling Pavilion (Park hrs)
Dovedale Sports Centre (Centre hrs)
Hylands Park, by parking area (Daytime)
Lionmead Park, Sandford Road (Daytime)
Melbourne Park, parking area (Daytime)

Moulesham Street/Hamlet Road
Oaklands Park (Park hrs)
Shopmobility, Market Road (Daytime)
Waterloo Lane, by Pool
The Meadows Shopping Centre *(Private)*
Sainsbury's Store, Springfield *(Sainsbury)*
Chelmsford Station *(NX East Anglia)*
Ladbrokes, Clematis Tye *(Ladbrokes)*
'Baroosh Restaurant', Moulsham Rd *(Private)*
'The Fleece', Duke Street *(Private)*
'Ivory Peg', New London Road *(JDW)*
'Nandos', Springfield Road *(Nandos)*
'Que Pasa', Springfield Rd *(Marstons)*
'Thomas Mildmay', Springfield Road *(JDW)*
Ashby House, Bishop Hall Road *(Anglia Ruskin University)*
Odeon Cinema, Kings Head Walk *(Odeon)*
Tenpin, Widford Industrial Estate *(Private)*

Danbury	Main Road, by Cricket Ground
Galleywood	Watchouse Road (Daytime)
Writtle	The Green (Daytime) 'Horse & Groom' *(Private)*
Woodham Ferrers	by Railway Station (Daytime) South Woodham Ferrers Leisure Centre (Centre hrs) Starz Youth Centre (Centre hrs) *(Essex CC)* William de Ferrers Adult Educ. Centre *(Essex CC)*

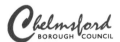

BOROUGH COUNCIL

Visit Chelmsford for quality
shopping opportunities.
It has a vibrant Market and
there is a Shopmobility Scheme
available.

Colchester

For information on disabled facilities in the area please call:
01206 282 700

Colchester

Colchester	Castle Park, by Boating Lake
	Castle Park, behind Hollytrees
	Cemetery, Mersea Road
	High Woods Country Park
	Queen Street Bus Station
	St John's Street MSCP
	St Mary's MSCP, Balkerne Hill
	Colchester Library (Library hrs) *(Essex CC)*
	Sir Isaac's Walk *(Private)*
	Osborne Street MSCP *(Private)*
	Colchester Station *(NX East Anglia)*
	'Nandos', Head Street *(Nandos)*
	'The Playhouse', St John Street *(JDW)*
	'Yates's Bar', Head Street *(Yates)*
	Gala Bingo, Osborne Street *(Gala)*
Dedham	Driftway
Great Horkesley	'Yew Tree' *(Private)*
Tiptree	Church Road

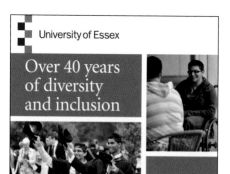

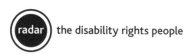

West Mersea	Coast Road Car Park High Street Victoria Esplanade (M+F)
Wivenhoe	High Street Car Park Sports Pavilion, Wivenhoe Park *(Essex University)* Students Union *(Essex University)* Sub Zero *(Essex University)*

Dacorum

Apsley	Durrants Hill Road
Berkhamstead	Water Lane Car Park, off High Street 'The Crown', High Street *(JDW)* 'Old Mill', London Road *(Private)*
Hemel Hempstead	Gadebridge Park King George V Car Park Market Square Bus Station Woodwells Cemetery (Cemetery hrs) Marlowes Shopping Centre *(Private)* Nash Mills Boat Base (Summer) *(Private)* 'The Full House', The Marlowes *(JDW)*
Kings Langley	High Street
Ringshall	Ashridge Estate, by Visitor Centre *(National Trust)*
Tring	Market Place Car Park, High Street

East Cambridgeshire

Ely	Barton Road Car Park (8.00-18.00) Cloisters Shopping Centre (8.00-18.00) Newnham Street Car Park Sacrist Gate, by Cathedral (8.00-18.00) Ship Lane Car Park, Riverside Ely Station, Platform 1 *(NX East Anglia)*
Littleport	Main Street Car Park (8.00-17.00)
Soham	Fountain Lane Car Park (7.30-19.30)
Wicken Fen	Lode Lane Car Park, near Nature Reserve Wren Building *(National Trust)*

East Hertfordshire

Bishops Stortford	Castle Gardens (April-October)
	Riverside Walk *(Town Council)*
	Bishops Stortford Station, Platform 1 *(NX East Anglia)*
Buntingford	Bowling Green Lane
Hertford	Bircherley Green, nr. Bus Station
	Hartham Common
	Hertford East Station *(NX East Anglia)*
	'Six Templars', The Wash *(JDW)*
Sawbridgeworth	Bell Street Car Park
Spellbrook	'Three Horseshoes', Spellbrook Lane *(Private)*
Ware	Priory Street *(Town Council)*

Epping Forest

Epping	Bakers Lane Car Park
High Beech	by Information Centre *(City of London)*
Hoddesdon	Dobbs Weir Car Park *(Lee Valley RPA)*
Loughton	Brook Path, High Road
	Traps Hill Car Park
	The Broadway *(Town Council)*
	'The Last Post', High Road *(JDW)*
Ongar	High Street

Waltham Abbey	Quaker Lane Car Park
	Fishers Green Car Park *(Lee Valley RPA)*
	High Bridge Street *(Town Council)*
	'Bakers Arms', Stewardstone Road *(Private)*

Fenland

Chatteris	Furrowfields
	Station Street
March	Broad Street
	City Road Car Park
Whittlesey	Eastgate Car Park
	Station Road
	'George Hotel', Market Place *(JDW)*
Wisbech	Church Terrace Car Park
	Exchange Square
	Wisbech Park
	Horsefair Shopping Centre *(Private)*
	'Wheatsheaf Inn', Church Terrace *(JDW)*

Forest Heath

Brandon	Brandon Country Park *(Suffolk CC)*
Lakenheath	Wings Road (07.00-19.00)
Mildenhall	Recreation Way
Newmarket	Memorial Gardens, High Street
	'Golden Lion', High Street *(JDW)*

Great Yarmouth

Caister	Beach Road Car Park (Easter-October)
	High Street
	Second Avenue (Easter-October)
	Yarmouth Stadium (Stadium hrs) *(Private)*
	Grasmere Caravan Park *(Private)*
Gorleston	Brush Quay
	High Street, opp. The Feathers
	Pier Head, by Ocean Rooms
	Ravine Bridge, Marine Parade
Great Yarmouth	Alpha Road/Southtown Road
	Caister Road/Beaconsfield Road

	The Conge, off Market Place The Jetty, Marine Parade Marina Beach (Easter-Oct, daytime) Market Gates (M+F) (9.00-17.00) North Beach, Seafront (8.00-18.30) The Tower, Marine Parade Great Yarmouth Station *(NX East Anglia)* 'The Troll Cart', Regent Road *(JDW)* Great Yarmouth Racecourse Caravan Site *(Caravan Club)* Vauxhall Holiday Park (2) *(Private)*
Hemsby	Beach Road (Easter-October)
Martham	Village Green
Winterton	Beach Car Park (Easter-Oct)

Harlow

Harlow	Bus Station, Terminus Street Bush Fair London Road, Old Harlow Shopmobility Car Park Staple Tye, by Shopping Precinct (M+F) (Daytime) The Stow, by Car Park Town Park, Greyhound Car Park Town Park, Pets Corner Harlow Town Station, Ticket Hall *(NX East Anglia)* 'Nandos', The Water Gardens *(Nandos)* 'William Aylmer', Kitson Way *(JDW)* 'Yates's Bar', Eastgate *(Yates)*

Hertsmere

Borehamwood	Station Road 'Hart & Spool', Shenley Road *(JDW)* Gala Bingo, Boulevard Park *(Gala)*
Bushey	King George Recreation Ground Rudolph Road
Potters Bar	Oakmere Park, High Street 'Admiral Byng', Darkes Lane *(JDW)*
Radlett	Radlett Station, Platform 4 *(Capital Connect)*
Shenley	London Road

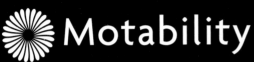

Motability

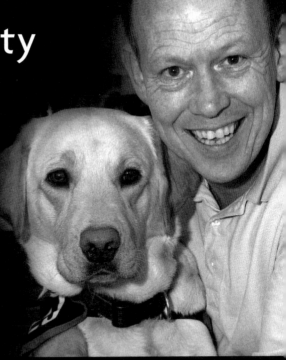

it changed our lives!

"Motability allows me to live life to the full. Just knowing you've got that backup 24 hours a day is real peace of mind."

Allen Parton and his assistance dog, EJ

where will yours take you?

use your mobility allowance to get mobile...

Simply exchange it for an all-inclusive worry-free mobility package, including:

- New car, powered wheelchair or scooter
- Insurance
- Servicing and repairs
- Tyres
- Breakdown cover

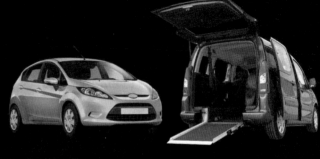

freephone
0800 093 1000

or visit www.motability.co.uk for further details

MO157C

Huntingdonshire

Godmanchester	School Hill/Post Street
Grafham Water	Mander Car Park *(Anglia Water)*
	Grafham Water Caravan Club Site *(Caravan Club)*
Huntingdon	Benedict's Court, Waitrose Complex
	Bus Station [To be redeveloped]
	Hinchingbrooke Country Park
	Riverside Pavilion, Hartford Road
	Grammar School Walk Car Park *(Private)*
	Shopmobility Centre, Princess St Car Park *(Shopmobility)*
	'Cromwells Bar', High Street *(Marstons)*
Ramsey	New Street/Great Whyte [To be redeveloped]
St Ives	Bus Station, Station Road/Cattlemarket
	West Street Car Park, Globe Place
St Neots	Riverside Park, Car Park
	Tebbuts Road, Car Park

Ipswich

Ipswich	Alexandra Park (Park hrs)
	Bourne Park, by Depot (Park hrs)
	Chantry Park, Hadleigh Road (Park hrs)
	Christchurch Park (3) (Park hrs)
	Holywell Park (Park hrs)
	Old Foundry Road
	Buttermarket Centre (2) *(Private)*

Tower Ramparts Centre *(Private)*
Ipswich Station *(NX East Anglia)*
Debenhams Store, Westgate St *(Debenhams)*
'The Cricketers', Crown Street *(JDW)*
'Nandos', Cardinal Leisure Park *(Nandos)*
'Old Orleans', Cardinal Park *(Private)*
'Robert Ransome', Tower Street *(JDW)*
CP Rushmere CRU (Centre hrs)

King's Lynn & West Norfolk

Brancaster	Beach Car Park, Broads Lane
Downham Market	Wales Court, Bridge Street (Daytime)
	Downham Market Station, Platform 1 *(Capital Connect)*
Heacham	North Beach, Jubilee Road
	South Beach Road (7.00-17.00)
Hilgay	Quayside (Apr-Oct)
Holme	Beach Road
Hunstanton	Bowling Green (7.00-17.00)
	Bus Station, Westgate
	Central Promenade, Seagate
	Cliff Top, Light House Close
	Esplanade Gardens
	Seagate Road (April-October)
King's Lynn	Baker Lane Car Park (7.30-18.00)
	Bus Station
	Ferry Street Car Park (7.30-18.00)
	Gaywood Road (Daytime)
	The Walks, Broadwalk (7.00-17.00)
	Kings Lynn Station, off Platform 1 *(Capital Connect)*
	'The Globe', King Street *(JDW)*
	'Lattice House', Chapel Street *(JDW)*
	'Nandos', High Street *(Nandos)*
	Kings Lynn Campus, Front Block *(W Anglia College)*
Sandringham	Sandringham Country Park *(Private)*
	Sandringham Caravan Club Site *(Caravan Club)*
Snettisham	Snettisham Beach

Luton

Luton	Burr Street, High Town
	Church Street, by Arndale Centre
	The Hat Factory (Centre hrs)
	Old Bedford Road, Wardown Park
	Purley Centre, Purway Close
	Sundon Park Road, Hill Rise
	The Mall Luton, Cheapside Square *(Private)*
	The Mall Luton, Market Hall *(Private)*
	Debenhams Store, The Mall *(Debenhams)*
	Marks & Spencer Store, The Mall *(M&S)*
	Luton Station, Platforms 3/4 *(Capital Connect)*
	Luton Parkway Station *(Capital Connect)*
	'Nandos', Galaxy Centre *(Nando)*
	'White House', Bridge Street *(JDW)*

Maldon

Burnham-on-Crouch	Doctor's Lane, The Quay (Daytime)
	Riverside Park
Heybridge	Bentalls Shopping Centre *(Private)*
Maldon	Butt Lane Car Park
	Promenade Coach Park
	Promenade Park Sea Wall
	Kings Head Centre *(Private)*
Tollesbury	Woodrolfe Road

Mid Suffolk

Barham	Barham Picnic Site *(Suffolk CC)*
Bramford	Picnic Site, Ship Lane *(Suffolk CC)*
Eye	Cross Street Car Park
Needham Market	The Lake
	Barratts Lane *(Town Council)*
Stowmarket	Milton Road Car Park
	Recreation Ground, Finborough Road *(Town Council)*
	Wilkes Way *(Town Council)*

North Hertfordshire

Ashwell	Ashridge Farm Caravan Club Site *(Caravan Club)*
Letchworth	Central Approach (Daytime) *(Private)* 'Three Magnets', Leys Avenue *(JDW)*

North Norfolk

Bacton	Coast Road
Blakeney	The Quay
Cromer	Cadogan Road Meadow Road Car Park/Information Centre Melbourne Pier Rocket House (Café hrs) Runton Road (mid-March – December) Seacroft Caravan Club Site *(Caravan Club)*
East Runton	Water Lane (March-December)
Fakenham	Bridge Street Highfields Queens Road Fakenham Racecourse Caravan Club Site *(Caravan Club)*
Happisburgh	Cart Gap (mid-March - Sept)
Hickling	Staithe
Holt	Albert Street Country Park
Horning	Swan Car Park
Hoveton	Station Road
Ludham	Ludham Bridge Womack Staithe Broadlands Caravan Club Site *(Caravan Club)*
Mundesley	Marina Road Promenade
North Walsham	New Road, Car Park
Overstrand	Pauls Lane Car Park (March – Dec and weekends)
Potter Heigham	Bridge
Sea Palling	Beach Road

Sheringham	East Promenade (March-October)
	High Street
	Station Approach
	West Promenade
	Sheringham Park *(National Trust)*
Stalham	High Street
Walcott	Coast Road
Walsingham	High Street
Wells-next-the-Sea	Newgate Lane
	Quay, Beach Road
West Runton	Incleboro Field Caravan Club Site *(Caravan Club)*

Norwich

Norwich	Chapelfield Gardens Park (Park hrs)
	Earlham Park (Park hrs)
	Eaton Park (Park hrs)
	Memorial Gardens, St Peter's Street (Mon-Sat)
	St Giles MSCP, St Giles Street
	St Saviours Lane (Mon-Sat)

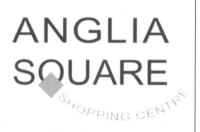

ANGLIA SQUARE
SHOPPING CENTRE

is pleased to support
Radar

ANGLIA SQUARE, NORWICH, NR3 1DZ

**A GREAT VARIETY OF STORES
AND SAFE PARKING**

Peterborough
City Council

Are pleased to
support the
Royal Association
for Disability Rights

Waterloo Park
Wensum Park (Apr-Oct, Park hrs)
Norwich Magistrates Court *(Courts Service)*
Anglia Square *(Private)*
The Mall Norwich (3) *(Private)*
Co-op Store, St Stephens Street *(Co-op)*
Debenhams Store, Orford Place *(Debenhams)*
Jarrolds Store, London Street *(Private)*
Norwich Station *(NX East Anglia)*
'Auberge', Castle Mall *(Private)*
'Bell Hotel', Orford Hill *(JDW)*
'Forget-me-Not Café', Redwell Street *(Private)*
'Glass House', Wensum Street *(JDW)*
'Ha! Ha! Bar', Tombland/Upper King St *(Private)*
'Henrys', Haymarket *(Private)*
'KFC', Dereham Road *(KFC)*
'KFC', Prince of Wales Road *(KFC)*
'Maid Marian', Ipswich Road *(Private)*
'Nandos', 23 Red Lion Street *(Nandos)*
'Nandos', 7b Riverside Leisure Park *(Nandos)*
'Norwegian Blue', Riverside Leisure Park *(Private)*
'Queen of Iceni', Riverside Leisure Park *(JDW)*
'Wagon & Horses', Dereham Road *(Private)*
'The Whiffler', Boundary Road *(JDW)*
Lower Common Room, UEA *(University)*
Cinema City, St Andrews Street *(Private)*
Hollywood Bowl, Riverside Leisure Park *(AMF)*
CP Whole Foodplanet, Yarefield Park *(Private)*

Peterborough

Peterborough

Car Haven Car Park (Daytime)
Northminster MSCP (Daytime)
St Peters Arcade, Bridge Street
Rivergate Shopping Centre *(Private)*
Peterborough Station, Platforms 2 & 5 *(East Coast)*
CP Mencap Business Support Centre, Hampton *(Mencap)*
'College Arms', The Broadway *(JDW)*
'Drapers Arms', Cowgate *(JDW)*
Peterborough Bowl, Sturrock Way, Bretton *(AMF)*
Ferry Meadows Caravan Club Site *(Caravan Club)*

Rochford

Ashingdon	Ashingdon Recreation Fields
	'Victory Inn', Ashingdon Rd *(Private)*
Great Wakering	High Street
Hockley	Hockley Road Car Park
	Hockley Woods Car Park
Hullbridge	Pooles Lane
Rayleigh	Crown Hill
	Warehouse Centre *(Private)*
	'Roebuck', High Street *(JDW)*
	'Travellers Joy', Down Hall Road *(Private)*
Rochford	Back Lane
	Rochford Station *(NX East Anglia)*
	'Anne Boleyn', Southend Road *(Private)*
Wallasea Island	Riverside Village Holiday Park *(Private)*

St Albans

Chiswell Green	'Three Hammers', Watford Road *(Private)*
Harpenden	'The George', High Street *(Private)*
London Colney	High Street (Daytime)
Redbourne	High Street Car Park
St Albans	Alban Arena, Foyer (Centre hrs)
	Alban Arena Car Park (M+F) (Daytime)
	Clarence Park, Bowling Green (Park hrs)
	Clarence Park, Ornamental Park (Park hrs)
	Drovers Way, Car Park
	Hatfield Road Cemetery (Cemetery hrs)
	Park Street
	The Ridgeway, Marshalswick, by Library
	Tourist & Information Centre, Town Hall (Centre hrs)
	Verulamium Park, Causeway (M+F)
	Verulamium Changing Rooms (M+F)
	Westminster Lodge Running Track
	The Maltings, off Victoria Street *(Private)*
	Jubilee Centre, Church Street *(Private)*
	'Cross Keys', Chequer Street *(JDW)*
	'Inn on the Park', Verulamium Park *(Private)*

	'Nandos', Chequer Street (*Nandos*)
	'Waterend Barn', St Peters Street (*JDW*)
Sandridge	High Street Car Park
Wheathampstead	East Lane Car Park
	'The Bull', High Street (*Beefeater*)

St Edmundsbury

Bury St Edmunds	Abbey Gardens, Angel Hill
	Bus Station
	Hardwick Heath, Hardwick Lane (8.30-dusk)
	Nowton Park
	Ram Meadow
	West Stow Country Park (Park hrs)
	Arc Shopping Centre (*Private*)
	Bury St Edmunds Station (*NX East Anglia*)
Clare	Clare Castle Country Park
Haverhill	Jubilee Walk
	Recreation Ground, Recreation Road
	Council Offices (Office hrs)
	'Drabbet Smock', Peas Hill (*JDW*)
Knettishall Heath	Knettishall Country Park (*Suffolk CC*)

South Cambridgeshire

| **Linton** | 'Dog & Duck' (*Private*) |
| **Milton** | Milton Country Park (*Private*) |

South Norfolk

Diss	Mere Mouth, behind TIC
Harleston	Bullock Fair Car Park
Hingham	Market Place
Loddon	Church Plain, High Street
Long Stratton	Swan Lane Car Park
Wymondham	Market Place

Southend-On-Sea

| **Chalkwell** | Chalkwell Esplanade, opp. Station |
| **CP** | Chalkwell Esplanade, opp Chalkwell Ave |

	Chalkwell Park, London Road
Leigh	Belfairs Park, Eastwood Road North
	Bell Wharf, Old Leigh High Street
	Eastwood Park, Rayleigh Road
	Elm Road, between Rectory Rd & Broadway
	Sutherland Boulevard/London Road
	Leigh-on-Sea Station, Concourse *(C2C)*
	'The Elms', London Road *(JDW)*
	'Sarah Moor', Elm Road *(Private)*
Prittlewell	'The Bell', Southend Arterial Road *(Private)*
Shoeburyness	George Street, East Beach Car Park
	Ness Road
	Shoebury Common, Car Park
	Shoebury Park, Elm Road
	Shoeburyness Station, Platform *(C2C)*
CP	Shoeburyness Leisure Centre *(Private)*
Southchurch	Southchurch Hall, Woodgrange Drive
	Southchurch Park, Liftsan Way
	'White Horse', Southchurch Road *(Private)*

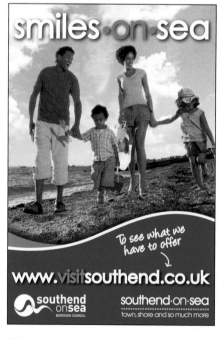

Southend	Dalmatia Road, nr. Southchurch Road
	Marine Parade, opp. The Ship
	Pitmans Close
	Priory Park, Victoria Avenue
	Seaway Car Park, Queensway (M+F)
	Pier Gardens (8.00-dusk) *(Private)*
	The Royals Shopping Centre *(Private)*
	Victoria Shopping Centre *(Private)*
	Debenhams Store, The Royals *(Debenhams)*
	Southend Central Station, Concourse *(C2C)*
	Southend East Station, Platform 1 *(C2C)*
	Southend Victoria Station *(NX East Anglia)*
	'Nandos', 24 London Road *(Nandos)*
	'Varsity', Chichester Road *(Barracuda)*
	Student Union, Elmer Approach *(University of Essex)*
	Mecca Bingo, Greyhound Shopping Park *(Mecca)*
	Odeon Cinema *(Odeon)*
	Roots Hall Stadium *(Southend Untd)*
Thorpe Bay	Thorpe Esplanade (Apr-October)
Westcliff	London Road/Hamlet Court Road
	Western Esplanade, by Café
	Westcliffe Station, Platform 2 *(C2C)*

Stevenage

Stevenage	Fairlands Valley Park, Sailing Centre
	Town Square
	Westgate Shopping Centre *(Private)*
	Stevenage Station, Concourse *(Capital Connect)*
	'KFC', Stevenage Leisure Park *(KFC)*
	'Nandos', Kings Way *(Nandos)*
	'The Proverbial', High Street *(Private)*
	'Standard Bearer', The Plaza *(JDW)*
	'The Standing Order', High Street *(JDW)*
	'White Lion', High Street *(Private)*

Suffolk Coastal

Aldeburgh	Fort Green
	Moot Hall
	West Lane
Bawdsey	The Ferry

Blythburgh	Toby's Walks Picnic Site *(Suffolk CC)*
Dunwich	Dunwich Beach
	Dunwich Heath, Coastguard Cottages *(National Trust)*
Felixstowe	Bathtap, Bath Hill
	Beach Station Road (Daytime)
	Crescent Road Car Park [2011]
	The Dip
	Golf Road Car Park
	Langer Park (Summer)
	Manor Road Car Park
	Ranelagh Road Car Park (Daytime)
	Spa Pavilion
	Town Hall
Framlingham	Crown & Anchor Lane
Leiston	Dinsdale Road (Daytime) *(Parish Council)*
	Sizewell Road (Daytime)
Martlesham	'Red Lion', Main Road *(Private)*
Orford	Quay Street Car Park *(Parish Council)*
Saxmundham	Market Place
Saxtead	The Green
Sizewell Beach	Car Park
Thorpeness	The Mere
Walberswick	Village
Wickham Market	Crafers Car Park (Daytime)

Woodbridge	Brook Street
	Elmhurst Park *(Parish Council)*
	Jetty Lane
	Station Road (Daytime)

Tendring

Brightlingsea	Promenade Way Car Park
	Station Road
	Waterside

Clacton	High Street Car Park
	Lower Promenade, Ambleside (Easter-Oct)
	Lower Promenade, West Greensward
	Magdalen Green, Old Road/Coppins Road
	Rosemary Road, opp. The Grove
	Westcliff, Middle Promenade, nr. Pier
	Clacton Station *(NX East Anglia)*
	'McDonalds', Pier Avenue *(Private)*
	'Moon & Starfish', Marine Parade East *(JDW)*
	Flicks Cinema, Pier Avenue *(Private)*
	Gala Bingo, Pier Avenue *(Private)*
Dovercourt	Cliff Park
	Low Road Playing Field
	Milton Road Car Park
	Wash Lane

Frinton	Greensward, Kiosk (May-Oct)
	Lower Promenade, opp. Cambridge Road
	Old Way

Harwich	by High Lighthouse, opp. George Street
Holland-on-Sea	Holland Gap, nr. Car Park
	Ipswich Road, nr. Car Park
	Middle Promenade, opp. Queensway (May-Oct)
	'Roaring Donkey', Holland Road *(Greene King)*
Jaywick	Meadow Way/Tamarisk Way
Manningtree	Market Site, Brook Street
Parkeston	Harwich Int. Station, Platform 1 *(NX East Anglia)*
Walton-on-the-Naze	Coronation Car Park, Princes Esplanade (May-Oct)
	Jubilee Beach, Lower Promenade (May-Oct)
	Mill Lane
	Pier Approach
	Walton-on-Naze Station *(NX East Anglia)*
	Walton Pier *(Private)*

Three Rivers

Rickmansworth	Aquadrome, Frogmoor Lane (Daytime)
	Three Rivers House, Northway
	'The Pennsylvanian', High Street *(JDW)*
South Oxhey	The Centre, Gosforth Lane

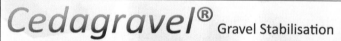

Thurrock

Aveley	Belhus Park Golf & Country Club *(Private)*
Chafford Hundred	Chafford Hundred Station, Booking Hall *(C2C)*
Grays	Grays Beach Riverside Park *(Private)*
	Grays Shopping Centre *(Private)*
	CP Grays Community Resource Centre
	Grays Station, Platform 1 *(C2C)*
	'Treacle Mine', Lodge Road *(Private)*
	Woodview Campus *(Thurrock & Basildon College)*
	Blackshots Leisure Centre, Blackshots Lane *(Private)*
Lakeside	Debenhams Store *(Debenhams)*
	'Las Iguanas', The Boardwalk *(Private)*
	'Nandos', Lakeside Pavilion *(Nandos)*
	'Wagamama', The Boardwalk *(Private)*
Little Thurrock	'Tyrrells Hall Club', Dock Road *(Private)*
North Stifford	'Dog & Partridge', High Road *(Private)*
Purfleet	'Royal Hotel', London Road *(Spirit)*
South Ockendon	**CP** South Ockendon Community Base (Office hrs)
Stanford-le-Hope	East Thurrock Community Association *(Private)*
	CP Stanford Base, The Sorrells
Tilbury	Tilbury Town Station, Platform 1 *(C2C)*
	'Anchor', Civic Square *(Private)*
	Tilbury Community Assn Leisure Centre *(Private)*
West Thurrock M25	Thurrock Services, J30/31 M25 *(Moto)*

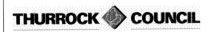

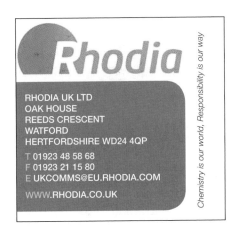

For more information on accessing public facilities in Thurrock, please telephone **01375 652 472** or email **diversity@thurrock.gov.uk**

RHODIA UK LTD
OAK HOUSE
REEDS CRESCENT
WATFORD
HERTFORDSHIRE WD24 4QP
T 01923 48 58 68
F 01923 21 15 80
E UKCOMMS@EU.RHODIA.COM
WWW.RHODIA.CO.UK

Chemistry is our world, Responsibility is our way

Uttlesford

Saffron Walden	The Common Car Park
	Swan Meadow
	'The Temeraire', High Street *(JDW)*
Stansted Airport	Terminal, Airside by Frankie & Bennies *(BAA)*
	Terminal, Airside by Wetherspoons *(BAA)*
	Terminal, Landside by O'Neills *(BAA)*
Stansted Mountfitchet	Lower Street Car Park

Watford

Garston	North Watford Cemetery (Cemetery hrs)
	Orbital Community Centre (Centre hrs)
	Watford Leisure Centre (2) (Centre hrs)
	Hollywood Bowl, Woodside Leisure Park *(AMF)*
Watford	Charter Place
	Cheslyn House, Nascoltwood Rd (Office hrs)
	Holywell Community Centre (Centre hrs)
	Watford Colosseum, Town Hall (Hall hrs)
	Harlequin Shopping Centre *(Private)*
	Watford Junction Station, Booking Hall *(London Midland)*
	'Bar Nazdarovya', 135 The Parade *(Private)*
	'Café Maximo Bar', High Street *(Private)*
	'Caffe Nero', High Street *(Caffe Nero)*
	'Chicago Rock Café', The Parade *(Private)*
	'Colombia Press', The Parade *(JDW)*
	'Destiny Night Club', The Parade *(Private)*
	'Essex Arms', Langley Way *(Private)*
	'The Flag', Station Road *(Private)*

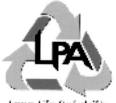
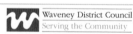

'Moon Under Water', High Street *(JDW)*
'Nando's', The Parade *(Nandos)*
'O'Neills', The Parade *(M&B)*
'Reflex', The Parade *(Private)*
'Revolution', High Street *(Private)*
'The Southern Cross', Langley Road *(Private)*
'Walkabout', High Street *(Private)*
Sportz Academy, The Parade *(Private)*
Vicarage Road Stadium *(Watford FC)*

Waveney

Beccles	Blyburgate Car Park
	Hungate Car Park
	Yacht Station, The Quay
Bungay	Priory Lane
Halesworth	Thoroughfare Car Park
Kessingland	Church Road
	Heathland Beach Caravan Park *(Private)*
	White House Beach Caravan Club Site *(Caravan Club)*
Lowestoft	Gordon Road
	Jubilee Parade North, South Beach (Summer)
	Kensington Gardens, A12
	Kirkley Cemetery
	Lowestoft Cemetery, Normanston Drive
	Pakefield Street
	Sparrow's Nest Park (Daytime)
	Triangle Market, High Street
Oulton Broad	Nicholas Everitt Park (Daytime)
Southwold	Church Green
	The Harbour, Ferry Road
	The Pier

Welwyn Hatfield

Hatfield	Galleria Shopping Centre (2) *(Private)*
	'Nandos', 66 Galleria *(Nandos)*
Welwyn Garden City	Stanborough Lakes, North
	Stanborough Lakes, South
	Howard Centre *(Private)*
	Commons Wood Caravan Club Site *(Caravan Club)*

Amber Valley

Alfreton	Bus Station, Severn Square
	Rogers Lane
	Cemetery, Rogers Lane (8.00-16.30)
	'Wagon & Horses', King Street *(JDW)*
	CP Genesis Family Entertainment Centre *(Private)*
Ambergate	Derby Road, A6/A610 junction
Belper	Belper Cemetery (Cemetery hrs)
	Bridge Street/Matlock Road, A6 Triangle
	River Gardens, Matlock Road
	Strutt Street
	The Firs Caravan Club Site *(Caravan Club)*
Codnor	Market Place
Crich	Browns Hill
Duffield	'Bridge Inn', Mareney Road *(Marstons)*
Heage	Eagle Street
Heanor	Market Place
	CP Shipley Country Park *(Derbys CC)*
	'Red Lion', Derby Road *(JDW)*
Holloway	Church Street
Lea Brooks	Cemetery (Cemetery hrs)

Ripley	Grosvenor Road
	Market Place
	'Red Lion', Market Place *(JDW)*
Somercotes	Market Place
	Sherwood Street Recreation Ground (8.00-16.30)
South Wingfield	Market Place

Ashfield

Hucknall	Market Place, Ogle Street
	'Bowman', Nottingham Road *(Private)*
	'Pilgrim Oak', High Street *(JDW)*
Huthwaite	Columbia Street
Kirkby-in-Ashfield	Station Street, Nags Head Street
Sutton-in-Ashfield	Idlewells Shopping Centre *(Private)*
	'The Picture House', Fox Street *(JDW)*

Bassetlaw

Blyth A1(M)	Blyth Services, A1M/A614 *(Moto)*
Clumber Park	Near Visitor Centre *(National Trust)*
	Cricket Ground *(National Trust)*
	Caravan Club Site *(Caravan Club)*
Retford	Bus Station waiting room (Station hrs)
	Chancery Lane (Shopping hrs)
	Chapelgate (Shopping hrs)
	Retford Station, Platform 1 *(East Coast)*

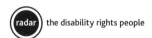 the disability rights people

Visit Radar's online shop

For a range of products to promote independent living.

www.radar-shop.org.uk

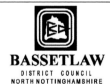

BASSETLAW
DISTRICT COUNCIL
NORTH NOTTINGHAMSHIRE

For information on Bassetlaw District Council public conveniences with access for the disabled, why not contact Environment Services?

Telephone Number
01909 534501

Visit: www.bassetlaw.gov.uk

'Broadstone' *(Private)*
'Dominie Cross', Grove Street *(JDW)*
'Hop Poles', Welham Road *(Private)*
'Litten Tree', Chapelgate *(Private)*
'Top House', Market Place *(Private)*

Worksop	Gateford Road (Shopping hrs)
	Park Street, Market (Shopping hrs)
	Priory Shopping Centre (Shopping hrs)
	The Hub, Memorial Avenue (Centre hrs)
	The Crossing Centre, Victoria Ave *(Private)*
	Worksop Station *(Northern Rail)*
	'Half Moon' *(Private)*
	'Liquorice Gardens', Newcastle Street *(JDW)*
	'Litten Tree', Victoria Square *(Private)*
	'Lock Keeper' *(Private)*
	'Three Legged Stool' *(Private)*
	'Top House' *(Private)*
	'White Lion' *(Private)*

Blaby

Blaby	John's Court, Waitrose Car Park
Glen Parva	'Glen Parva Manor', The Ford *(Marstons)*
Kirby Muxloe	'Castle Hotel', Main Street *(Private)*

Bolsover

Bolsover		Cavendish Walk (Mon-Sat, daytime)
Shirebrook	**CP**	Carter Lane Day Centre (Centre hrs)

Boston

Boston		Cattle Market Car Park, Bargate
		Central Park (Park hrs)
		Lincoln Lane
		Market Place (Daytime)
		'Moon Under Water', High Street *(JDW)*
	CP	Princess Royal Sports Arena (Centre hrs)
Leverton		Picnic Area, off A52 (M+F)

Broxtowe

Beeston	Beeston Fields Recreation Ground
	Broadgate Park, High Road
	Bus Station
	Leyton Crescent Recreation Ground
	Weirfields Recreation Ground, Canal Side
	'Last Post', Chilwell Road *(JDW)*
Chilwell	'Charlton Arms', High Road *(Private)*
Eastwood	Nottingham Road, by Library
Kimberley	Main Street
Stapleford	Ilkeston Road Recreation Ground
	Queen Elizabeth Park, Toton Lane
	The Roach
Toton	Manor Farm Recreation Ground

Charnwood

Anstey	The Nook Car Park (8.00-18.00)
Barrow-on-Soar	High Street Car Park (8.00-18.00)
Birstall	Stonehill Avenue (8.00-18.00)
Loughborough	Beehive Lane
	Biggin Street
	Charnwood Water (8.00-18.00)
	Granby Street
	Market Yard (8.00-18.00)
	Outwoods Park (Park Events)
	Queens Park (8.00-18.00)
	Southfield Park (Park Events)
	Sainsbury's Store, Greenclose La. *(Sainsbury)*
	'Amber Rooms', The Rushes *(JDW)*
	'Moon & Bell', Wards End *(JDW)*
	'Varsity', Market Street *(Barracuda)*
Markfield M1	Leicester Services, A50/M1 *(Moto)*
Shepshed	Hallcroft (8.00-18.00)
Sileby	King Street (8.00-18.00)
Syston	Melton Road (8.00-18.00)
Woodhouse Eaves	Main Street (8.00-18.00)

Chesterfield

Brimington	High Street
Chesterfield	Beetwell Street Coach Station
	New Square, Market Hall Basement (Mon-Sat, daytime)
	Pavements Centre (Mon-Sat, daytime)
	Queens Park, North Lodge (Daytime)
	Vicar Lane Shopping Centre *(Private)*
	Sainsbury's Store, Rother Way *(Sainsbury)*
	Chesterfield Station, Platform 1 *(E. Midlands Trains)*
	'Portland Hotel', West Bars *(JDW)*
	'Spa Lane Vaults', St Marys Gate *(JDW)*
	'Yates's Bar', Burlington Street *(Yates)*
Hollingwood	'Hollingwood Hotel', Private Drive *(Marstons)*
Newbold	Holmebrook Valley Park (dawn-dusk)
Old Whittington	by Swanick Memorial Hall, High Street
Somersall	Somersall Park, Somersall Lane
Staveley	Market Place Car Park
	Poolsbrook County Park, Fan Rd (dawn-dusk)
	Poolsbrook Caravan Club Site *(Caravan Club)*

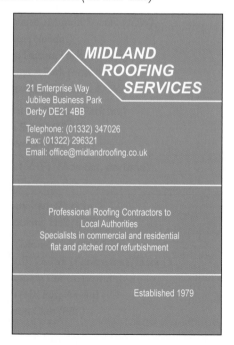

Tapton	Tapton Park (Dawn-dusk)
Whittington Moor	Duke Street, off Sheffield Road

Corby

Corby	Boating Lake, Cottingham Road (Park hrs)
	CP Corby International Swimming Pool (Pool hrs)
	Market Walk, Queens Square *(Private)*
	Willow Place Shopping Centre *(Private)*
	'Samuel Lloyd', Rockingham Rd/Gretton Rd *(JDW)*
	CP Civic Hub Shopping Complex [Planned]
East Carlton	East Carlton Countryside Park (Park hrs)

Daventry

Daventry	Daventry Country Park, Welton Road
	New Street, by Bus Station
	'Queen of Hearts', Ashby Fields *(Marstons)*
	'Saracen's Head', Brook Street *(JDW)*

Derby

Derby	Allenton Market (Market hrs
	Arboretum, Rosehill Street end
	Bold Lane Car Park
	Chaddesdon Park, Chaddesdon Lane
	Darley Park, nr. Café
	Darley Playing Fields
	Eagle Centre Market (Market hrs)
	Markeaton Park, nr Craft Village
	Markeaton Park Island, Ashbourne Road
	Market Hall Balcony
	Market Place, opp. Tourist Information (8.00-17.00)
	Munday Play Centre
	Park Farm Centre, Allentree
	Rowditch Recreation Ground
	The Spot, London Road/Osmaston Road (8.00-17.00)
	Victoria Street (8.00-17.00)
	Wade Street/Burton Road
	CP Westfield Shopping Centre *(Private)*
	Derby Station, Platforms 1 & 4 *(E Midlands Trains)*
	'Babington Arms', Babington Lane *(JDW)*
	'Fat Cat Café Bar', Friar Gate *(Private)*

'Nandos', 15 Market Place *(Nandos)*
'Nandos', Westfield Centre *(Nandos)*
'Revolution', Wardwick *(Private)*
'Soda Bar', Friar Gate *(Private)*
'Standing Order', Irongate *(JDW)*
'Varsity', Friar Gate *(Private)*
'Walkabout', Market Place *(Private)*
College Reception, Prince Charles Ave *(Derby College)*
Design Centre, Prince Charles Ave. *(Derby College)*
Sports Centre, Prince Charles Ave. *(Derby College)*
Gala Bingo, Foresters Leisure Park *(Gala*
Gala Bingo, Liversage Road *(Gala)*
Pride Park Stadium *(Derby County FC)*

Derbyshire Dales

Ashbourne	Bus Station Recreation Ground Shaw Croft Car Park
Ashford-in-the-Water	[No specific information available]
Bakewell	Agricultural Business Centre (Centre hrs) Granby Road Recreation Ground Riverside
Baslow	[No specific information available] Chatsworth Park Caravan Club Site *(Caravan Club)*
Bradwell	[No specific information available]
Cromford	Memorial Gardens
Darley Dale	Station Road
Dovedale	Dovedale Car Park *(Peak District NP)*
Eyam	[No specific information available]
Hartington	[No specific information available]
Hathersage	[No specific information available]
Kirk Ireton	Blackwall Plantation Caravan Club Site *(Caravan Club)*
Matlock	Artists Corner Bus Station Hall Leys Play Area Hall Leys Roadside

	'The Crown', Crown Square *(JDW)*
Matlock Bath	North Parade
	Pavilion
Middleton-by-Youlgreave	[No specific information available]
Middleton Top	Picnic Site *(Derbys CC)*
Monsal	Monsal Head
Over Haddon	[No specific information available]
Parsley Hay	Cycle Hire Centre, A515 *(Private)*
Stannage	Hollin Bank Car Park *(Peak District NP)*
Thorpe	[No specific information available]
Tideswell	[No specific information available]
	Tideswell Dale Car Park *(Peak District NP)*
White Lodge	White Lodge Car Park *(Peak District NP)*
Winster	[No specific information available]
Wirksworth	Barmcote Croft Car Park

East Lindsey

Alford	South Market Place Car Park
Anderby	Anderby Creek
Burgh Le Marsh	Market Place
Chapel St Leonards	Bus Station, Sea Road (Daytime)
	Chapel Point (Easter-October)
	Trunch Lane (Easter-October)
Conningsby	Car Park, off High Street
Horncastle	St Lawrence Street (Daytime)
	CP Horncastle Swimming Pool (Pool hrs)
Huttoft	Huttoft Bank
Ingoldmells	Sea Lane, Beach Bar (Summer, daytime)
Louth	Bus Station, Church Street (Daytime)
	Eastgate, by Market Hall (Daytime)
	Hubbards Hill (Daytime)
	Newmarket (Daytime)
	CP Meridian Leisure Centre (Centre hrs)
Mablethorpe	Central Promenade (Summer, daytime)

		Dunes Gardens, Quebec Road (Daytime) Golf Road (Summer, daytime) North End (Summer, daytime) Queens Park (Easter-Oct & weekends) Seacroft Road Bus Station (Daytime) Seaview Car Park (Summer, Daytime) South Promenade (Summer, Daytime)
North Somercotes		Playing Field
North Thoresby		[No specific information available] (Daytime)
Saltfleet		Sea Lane (Daytime)
Skegness	**CP**	Briar Way (Daytime) Lumley Square (Daytime) North Parade (Summer, daytime) Princes Parade (Summer, daytime) Tower Esplanade (Daytime) Tower Gardens (Daytime) Skegness Station *(E. Midlands Trains)* 'Red Lion', Roman Bank *(JDW)* Embassy Centre, Upper Foyer *(Private)*
Spilsby		Market Place (Daytime)
Sutton-on-Sea		Bohemia (Daytime) by Sandilands Golf Course (Daytime) Sutton Pleasure Gardens (Daytime) Hawthorn Farm Caravan Club Site *(Caravan Club)*
Tetney		by Village Hall (Daytime)
Wainfleet		Brooks Walk (6.00-20.00)
Winthorpe		Sandfield, Roman Bank (Summer, daytime) Winthorpe Avenue (Summer, daytime)
Woodhall Spa		Jubilee Park (Easter-October) Spa Road (Daytime)
Wragby		Market Place (Daytime)

East Northamptonshire

Higham Ferrers	Wharf Road (Daytime)
Irthlingborough	High Street (Daytime)
Oundle	St Osyth's Lane (Daytime)
Raunds	Marshalls Road *(Town Council)*

Rushden	Duck Street (Daytime)
	Newton Road (Daytime)
Thrapston	Oundle Road (Daytime)

Erewash

Borrowash	Victoria Avenue, Supermarket Car Park
Breaston	Blind Lane
Draycott	Markets Street/Derby Street
Ilkeston	Gallows Inn
	Market Place, Bath Street
	Station Road
CP	Co-op Department Store, Market Place *(Co-op)*
	'Moon & Sixpence', Woodland Ave *(Private)*
	'The Observatory', Market Place *(JDW)*
Long Eaton	Hall Grounds
	Orchard Street
	Long Eaton Station
	Trent Lock
	West Park Pavilion
	'Twitchel Inn', Howitt Street *(JDW)*

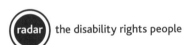

radar) the disability rights people

Become a member of Radar

Network with like-minded people
and keep up to date with disability
sector news.

www.radar.org.uk

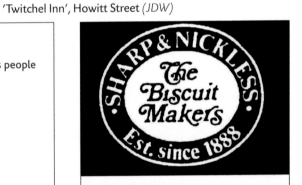

Sandiacre	Longmoor Lane
Sawley	'Bell Inn', Tamworth Road *(Private)*
Trowell M1	Trowell Services, J25/26 M1 *(Moto)*

Gedling

Arnold	Arnot Hill Park (Kiosk hrs)
	Burntstump Park Car Park (8.00-17.00)
	Front Street
	Redhill Cemetery (Cemetery hrs)
	Wood Street (8.00-18.00)
	Methodist Church, Market Place *(Church)*
	'Burnt Stump', Burnt Stump Hill *(Marstons)*
	'The Ernehale', Nottingham Road *(JDW)*
	'Friar Tuck', Gedling Road *(Private)*
Bestwood Country Park	Alexandra Lodge *(Notts CC)*
Burton Joyce	Church Road
	'Wheatsheaf Inn', Main Street *(Private)*
Calverton	St Wilfreds Square (8.00-17.00)
Carlton	Albert Avenue
	Cavendish Road, nr. Cemetery (8.00-Dusk)
Gedling	'Chesterfield Arms', Main Road *(Private)*
Mapperley	Haywood Road Car Park
	'Woodthorpe Top', Woodthorpe Rd *(JDW)*
Ravenshead	Milton Court Shopping Precinct

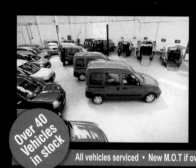

| Stoke Bardolph | 'Ferry Boat Inn'*(Private)* |

Harborough

Little Bowden	Recreation Ground
Lutterworth	George Street Car Park
Market Harborough	The Commons Car Park
	Welland Park, Welland Park Road
	Market Harborough Station, Platform 1 *(E Midlands Trains)*
	'Peacock', St Mary's Place *(Marstons)*
	'The Sugar Loaf'', High Street *(JDW)*

High Peak

Bamford	Main Road
Buxton	Market Place (8.00-17.00)
	Sylvan Car Park
	Grin Low Country Park *(Derbys CC)*
	'Wye Bridge House', Fairfield Road *(JDW)*
	Grin Low Caravan Club Site *(Caravan Club)*
Castleton	Losehill Caravan Club Site *(Caravan Club)*
Chinley	Green Lane
Crowden	Car Park *(Peak District NP)*
Edale	Car Park
Glossop	'Norfolk Arms', High Street *(Private)*
Hadfield	Platt Street
Hayfield	Sett Valley Trail Car Park *(Derbys CC)*
	Bowden Bridge Car Park *(Peak District NP)*
Hope	Castleton Road Car Park 99.00-17.00)
New Mills	High Street
Whaley Bridge	Market Street

Hinckley & Bosworth

Barwell	Top Town, Shilton Road (Daytime)
Hinckley	Ashby Road Cemetery (Cemetery hrs)
	Hollycroft Park Pavilion (Park hrs)
	Leisure Centre, Coventry Road (Centre hrs)
	Station Road (Daytime)

'Baron of Hinckley', Regent Street *(JDW)*

'Hinckley Knights', Watling Street *(Private)*

Newbold Verdon   Methodist Church Car Park *(Church)*

Kettering

Burton Latimer   Churchill Way Car Park

Kettering   Dalkeith Place

Ebenezer Place

Rockingham Park, Park Road

Newlands Shopping Centre *(Private)*

Kettering Station, Platform 1 *(E Midlands Trains)*

'Earl of Dalkeith', Dalkeith Place *(JDW)*

'Nandos', Kettering Business Park *(Nandos)*

CP The Shop, God Street *(Private)*

Rothwell   Squires Hill

Leicester

Leicester   Beaumont Leys Market

Belgrave Road, by Flyover

Charles Street Bus Station (Mon-Sat, 7.00-19.00)

Clarendon Gardens, by Library

Cossington Street, by Recreation Ground

East Park Road, Spinney Hill Park

Foundary Square, Belgrave Gate

Infirmary Square

Knighton Lane East, opp. Leisure Centre

Newark Street. By MSCP (Mon-Sat, 7.00-16.30)

Retail Market (Mon-Sat, 9.00-17.00)

St Margaret's Bus Station, Gravel Street

Welford Road, Nelson Mandela Park

Western Park, by play area

Leicester Station, Platforms 2 & 4 *(E. Midlands Trains)*

'Corn Exchange', Market Place *(JDW)*

'Gynsills', Leicester Road, Glenfield *(Private)*

'Heathley Park', Groby Road *(Private)*

'High Cross', High Street *(JDW)*

'Jongleurs', Granby Street *(Private)*

'Last Plantagenet', Granby Street *(JDW)*

'Nandos', Freemans Leisure Park *(Nandos)*

'Nandos', Granby Street *(Nandos)*

'Nandos', Highcross *(Nandos)*
'Owl & Pussycat', Melton Road *(Private)*
'Varsity', Friar Lane *(Barracuda)*
'Varsity', London Road *(Barracuda)*
'Walkabout', Granby Street *(Private)*
'Yates's Bar', Belvoir Street *(Yates)*
Bennett Building *(Univ of Leicester)*
Fielding Johnson Building *(Univ of Leicester)*
Fosse Neighbourhood Centre *(Leicester College)*
Walkers Stadium *(Leics City FC)*
CP High Cross Shopping Centre *(Private)*

Lincoln

Lincoln
Castle Square
City Bus Station
Hartsholme Country Park, Visitor Centre (Daytime)
Westgate, nr. Union Road
CP Yarborough Leisure Centre (Centre hrs)
Waterside Shopping Centre *(Private)*
Lincoln Station, Platform 5 *(E. Midlands Trains)*
'The Forum', Silver Street *(JDW)*
'Nandos', Brayford Wharf North *(Nandos)*
'The Ritz', High Street *(JDW)*
'Slug & Lettuce', Brayford Wharf *(Private)*
'Square Sail', Brayford Wharf North *(JDW)*
'Varsity', Guildhall Street *(Barracuda)*
'Walkabout', High Street *(Private)*

Mansfield

Mansfield
Bus Station
Four Seasons Shopping Centre
Mansfield Town Hall [to be refurbished]
Mansfield Library *(Notts CC)*
Mansfield Station *(E. Midlands Trains)*
'Courthouse', Market Place *(JDW)*
'Ravensdale', Sherwood Hall Rd *(Marstons)*
'Rufford', Chesterfield Rd South *(Marstons)*
'Rushley', Nottingham Road *(Marstons)*
'Stag & Pheasant', Clumber Street *(JDW)*
'Swan', Church Street *(Marstons)*
'Widow Frost', Leeming Street *(JDW)*

	'Yates's Bar', Leeming Street *(Yates)*
	Gala Bingo, Albert Street *(Gala)*
Mansfield Woodhouse	Rose Lane
Warsop	High Street Car Park

Melton

Melton Mowbray	Cattle Market (Market Days)
	Park Lane
	St Mary's Way
	'Kettleby Cross', Wilton Road *(JDW)*
	Mencap & Gateway Centre, Chapel St *(Mencap)*

Newark & Sherwood

Bilsthorpe	'Copper Beech', Kirklington Road *(Private)*
Clipstone	Vicar Water Country Park Visitor Centre (Daytime)
Edwinstowe	Mansfield Road, by Village Hall
	Sherwood Forest Country Park Visitor Centre *(Notts CC)*
Gunthorpe	'Anchor Inn', Main Street *(Private)*
	'Unicorn Hotel', Gunthorpe Bridge *(Private)*
Kelham	Kelham Hall Civic Suite (Suite hrs)
Laxton	Dovecote Inn Car Park (Dawn-Dusk)
Lowdham	Southwell Rd/Main Street
New Balderton	'The Grove', London Road *(Private)*
Newark	Castle Grounds, Gilstrap Building (Daytime)
	London Road Car Park (Daytime)

Sconce & Devon Park (Park hrs)
Tolney Lane, Riverside Park
Buttermarket *(Private)*
Newark Northgate Station, Platforms 1&3 *(East Coast)*
'Atrium', Castle Gate *(Private)*
'Sir John Arderne', Church Street *(JDW)*

Ollerton	Sherwood Heath Inf. Centre (Centre hrs)
Rainworth	'Robin Hood', Southwell Road East *(Private)*
Rufford	Rufford Abbey Country Park, The Abbey *(Notts CC)* 'Rose Cottage', Old Rufford Road *(Private)*
Southwell	Church Street Car Park

North East Derbyshire

Ashover	'Crispin Inn', Church Street *(Private)*
Clay Cross	Market Street *(Parish Council)*
Dronfield	Cliff Park, Calleywhite Lane *(Town Council)*
Grassmoor	'Boot & Shoe', North Wingfield Road *(Private)*

North East Lincolnshire

Cleethorpes	CP	Boating Lake, off Kings Road
		Kingsway, nr. Leisure Centre
		St Peter's Avenue, off Car Park
		Sea Road
		Cleethorpes Station *(Transpennine)*
		'The Wellow', Kings Road *(Private)*
		Pleasure Island *(Private)*

Grimsby		Garibaldi Street (Mon-Sat 8.30-17.30)
		Market Hall (Mon-Sat 8.30-17.30)
		Freshney Place Shopping Centre *(Private)*
		'Bradley Inn', Bradley Crossroads *(Private)*
		'DN31', Victoria Street *(Private)*
		'Ice Barque', Frederick Ward Way *(JDW)*
		'The Parity', Old Market Place *(Barracuda)*
		'Yarborough Hotel', Bethlehem St. *(JDW)*
		Great Grimsby Swimming Pool, Scartho Rd *(Private)*
		Grimsby Leisure Centre, Cromwell Rd *(Private)*
Immingham	CP	Town Council Offices, Pelham Way (Town Council)
Stallingborough		'Green Man', Station Road *(Private)*
Waltham		Waltham Windmill & Grounds
		'Kings Head', High Street *(Private)*

North Kesteven

North Hykeham	CP	North Keseven Leisure Centre (Centre hrs)
Sleaford		Money's Yard, Carre Street (8.00-17.00)
		'Packhorse Inn', Northgate *(JDW)*
Whisby		Whisby Nature Park, Visitor Centre *(Private)*

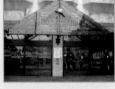

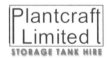

North Lincolnshire

Barton-on-Humber	Baysgarth Park, Caistor Road
	Humber Bridge Viewing Area
	Market Place
Belton	Picnic Area, off A161
Brigg	Barnard Avenue/Bigby High Road
	Cary Lane
	Elsham Country Park, Car Park *(Private)*
Epworth	Chapel Street Car Park
Haxey	Vinehall Road/High Street
Owston Ferry	High Street
Scunthorpe	Ashby Broadway, Car Park
	Dunstall Street Car Park
	Frodingham Road/Doncaster Road
	John Street MSCP
	Library Square MSCP
	Normanby Hall Country Park
	Normanby Hall Country Park, Car Park
	Parishes MSCP, by Shopmobility
	Scunthorpe Station *(Transpennine)*
	'Blue Bell Inn', Oswald Road *(JDW)*
	Scunthorpe Bowl, Warren Road *(Private)*

North West Leicestershire

Ashby-de-la-Zouch	Kilwardby Street/Derby Road
Coalville	Precinct (Mon-Sat, 7.30-18.00)
	'Monkey Walk', Marlborough Square *(JDW)*
Donnington Park M1	Donington Park Services, J23A M1 *(Moto)*
Moira	Moira Craft Workshops *(Private)*

Northampton

Northampton	Guildhall, St Giles Square (Office hrs)
	Central Library, Abington Street *(Northants CC)*
	Grosvenor Shopping Centre *(Private)*
	Peacock Place Shopping Centre *(Private)*
CP	Weston Favel Shopping Centre *(Private)*
	Debenhams Store, The Drapery *(Debenhams)*

Greyfriars Bus Station *(Private)*
Northampton Station, Booking Hall *(London Midland)*
'Ask'', St Giles Square *(Private)*
'Auctioneers', Market Square *(Marstons)*
'Billing Mill Restaurant', The Causeway *(Private)*
'Chicago Rock Café', Market Square *(Private)*
'Cordwainer', The Ridings *(JDW)*
'Fish Inn', Fish Street *(Private)*
'Fox & Hounds', Harborough Rd, Kingsthorpe *(Private)*
'Frog & Fiddler', Harborough Road *(Private)*
'Hart of Dunston', Harlestone Rd, Dunston *(Private)*
'Hungry Horse', Sixfields Leisure Park *(Private)*
'KFC', Marquee Drive *(KFC)*
'Lloyds Bar', Abington Street *(JDW)*
'Moon on the Square'', Market Square *(JDW)*
'N.B's', Bridge Street *(Private)*
'Queen Eleanor', London Road, Wootton *(Private)*
'Toad at Sol Central', Sol Central *(Private)*
'White Elephant', Kingley Park Terrace *(Private)*
Billings Aquadrome *(Private)*
Tenpin 10, Sixfields Leisure Park *(Private)*
CP Pitsford Sports Arena *(Moulton College)*

Nottingham

Nottingham   Duke Street, Bulwell (7.00-18.00)
CP Greyhound Street, Market Square .
CP Djanogley Community Leisure Centre, Gregory Boulevard
Gregory Boulevard, Hyson Green (7.00-18.00)

CP Ken Martin Leisure Centre, Bulwell (Centre hrs)
CP Mary Potter Centre, Hyson Green (Centre hrs)
Spondon Street, Sherwood
Trent Bridge, Victoria Embankment
CP Wollaton Hall, Wollaton Park
Debenhams Store, Long Row *(Debenhams)*
Nottingham Station, Platforms 1&5 *(E. Midlands Trains)*
'Broxtowe Inn', Nuthall Rd, Cinderhill *(Private)*
'Company Inn', Castle Wharf *(JDW)*
'Fox', Valley Road, Basford *(Private)*
'Free Man' Carlton Hill *(JDW)*
'Grove Castle Hotel', Castle Boulevard *(Private)*
'Ha! Ha! Bar', Weekday Cross *(Private)*
'Jongleurs', Castle Wharf *(Private)*
'Joseph Else', Market Square *(JDW)*
'KFC', Lower Parliament Street *(KFC)*
'Liit Nottingham', Market Street *(Private)*
'Lloyds Bar', Carlton Street *(JDW)*
'Nandos', Angel Row, Market Sq *(Nandos)*
'Nandos', Redfield Way, Lenton *(Nandos)*
'Old Dog & Partridge', Lower Parliament St *(Private)*
'Pit & Pendulum', Victoria Street *(Private)*
'Roebuck Inn', St James Street *(JDW)*
'Samuel Hall', Old Bus Depot, Sherwood *(JDW)*
'Varsity', Peel Street *(Barracuda)*
'Walkabout'', Friar Lane *(Private)*
'Willoughby Arms', Wollaton *(Private)*
Carlton Road Centre *(Castle College)*

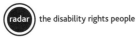 **radar** the disability rights people

Get Motoring

Your guide to everything the disabled motorist needs to know about finding, financing and maintaining a car.

Available from Radar's online shop
www.radar-shop.org.uk

Nottingham City Council

For more information on Public Facilities and Access at many attractions, why not telephone for more details before you travel?

Please telephone
0115 915 5330
for all enquiries

Gala Bingo, Hucknell Road *(Gala)*
Gala Bingo, St Ann's Well Road *(Gala)*
CP Nottingham Contemporary Arts Centre (Centre hrs)

Oadby & Wigston

Great Glen	'Yews', London Road *(Private)*
Oadby	East Street Car Park
	'Horse & Hounds', Glen Rise *(Private)*
	'Lord Keeper of the Great Seal', The Parade *(JDW)*
South Wigston	Blaby Road
Wigston	Junction Road
	Peace Memorial Park
	'William Wygston', Leicester Road *(JDW)*

Rushcliffe

Ruddington	'Millers', Loughborough Road *(Private)*
Wilford	'Ferry Inn' *(Private)*
West Bridgford	Bridgford Park, Central Avenue (Dawn-dusk)

Rutland

Oakham	**CP**	Church Street Car Park (7.00-18.00)
		John Street, Westgate Car Park (7.00-18.00)
Uppingham		Market Place (7.00-18.00)

South Derbyshire

Etwall	Eggington Road (Dawn-dusk)
Melbourne	Leisure Centre *(Private)*
Overseal	Woodsville Road (Dawn-dusk)
Repton	'Bulls Head', High Street *(Private)*
Shardlow	'Clock Warehouse' *(Marstons)*
Swadlincote	Bus Park, Civic Way (Dawn-dusk)
	East End Car Park (Dawn-dusk)
	'Sir Nigel Gresley', Market Street *(JDW)*
Ticknall	Ingleby Lane (Dawn-dusk)
	Calke Abbey, Restaurant Yard *(Nat. Trust)*
Willington	Canal Bridge (Dawn-dusk)

South Holland

Crowland	Town Centre
	West Street
Donnington	Park Lane, off A52
Holbeach	Church Street
Long Sutton	West Street
Spalding	Ayscoughfee Gardens (8.00-dusk)
	Bus Station, Winfrey Avenue
	Sheepmarket (8.00-18.00)
	Vine Street
	'Ivy Wall', New Road *(JDW)*
Sutton Bridge	Bridge Road, off A17

South Kesteven

Bourne		South Street *(Town Council)*
Deeping St James	**CP**	Deeping Leisure Centre (Centre hrs)
Gonerby Moor A1		Grantham North Services, A1 *(Moto)*
Grantham		Abbey Gardens
		Arnoldfield Playing Field (Apr-Sept, 9.00-19.00)
		Conduit Lane
		London Road
		George Shopping Centre *(Private)*
		Grantham Station, Platform 1 *(East Coast)*
		'Tollemache Inn', St Peter's Hill *(JDW)*
		Gala Bingo, Trent Road *(Gala)*
Market Deeping		The Precinct *(Town Council)*
Stamford		Red Lion Square

South Northamptonshire

Brackley	Market Place
Stoke Bruerne	'Navigation', Bridge Road *(Marstons)*
Towcester	Sponne Precinct Car Park, Richmond Road

Wellingborough

Finedon	Recreation Ground, Wellingborough Road
Sywell	'Overstone Manor', Ecton Lane *(Private)*
Wellingborough	Bassetts Park
	Commercial Way MSCP (2) (7.30-17.30)
	Embankment
	Market Square (7.30-18.00)
	Swanspool Gardens (7.30-dusk)
	Wellingborough Station, Platform 1 *(E Midlands Trains)*
	'Red Well', Silver Street *(JDW)*
	Wellingborough Bowl, Victoria Retail Pk *(AMF)*
	CP Waendel Leisure Centre (Centre hrs)

West Lindsey

Caistor	Town Hall Car Park
Gainsborough	Corporation Yard, Bridge Street [Under construction]
	Roseway Car Park
	Whittons Gardens, Caskgate Street
	'Sweyn Forkbeard', Silver Street *(JDW)*
Market Rasen	Willingham Wood, by Café, A631

West Lindsey District Council

For more information on Public Facilities and Access at many attractions, why not telephone for more details before you travel?

Please telephone for all enquiries: 01427 676 676

---

 the disability rights people

Get Mobile

Radar's independent guide to help you purchase a mobility scooter or powered wheelchair.

Available from Radar's online shop
www.radar-shop.org.uk

Birmingham

Acocks Green	Westley Road, by Laffertys
	'Spread Eagle', Warwick Road *(JDW)*
Aston	Villa Park *(Aston Villa FC)*
Birmingham City Centre	Central Library (Library hours)
	Hurst Street/Queensway
	Newton Street
	Steelhouse Lane
	Stephenson Place
	Waterloo Street
	Millennium Point, Curzon Street *(Private)*
	Pallasades Shopping Centre *(Private)*
	Pavilion Central, by Food Court *(Private)*
	Moor Street Station *(Chiltern Railway)*
	New Street Station, Concourse *(Network Rail)*
	Snow Hill Station, Platforms *(London Midland)*
	'Briar Rose', Bennetts Hill *(JDW)*
	'Dragon Inn', Hurst Street *(JDW)*
	'Figure of Eight', Broad Street *(JDW)*
	'Ha! Ha! Bar', The Mailbox *(Private)*
	'The Hornet', Alum Rock Road *(JDW)*
	'Jongleurs', Quayside Tower *(Private)*
	'Malt House', Brindley Place *(Private)*
	'Nandos', The Mailbox *(Nandos)*
	'Nandos', R2 The New Bullring *(Nandos)*
	'Nandos', Paradise Forum *(Nandos)*
	'Old Joint Stock', Temple Row West *(Fullers)*
	'Old Orleans', Broad Street *(Private)*
	'Soloman Cutler', Regency Wharf *(JDW)*
	'Square Peg', Corporation Street *(JDW)*
	'Toad at the Bullring', Hurst Street *(Private)*
	'Walkabout', Regency Wharf *(Private)*
	'Wetherspoons', Paradise Place *(JDW)*
	Gala Casino, Hill Street *(Gala)*
Cotteridge	Pershore Road, opp Watford Road
Digbeth	Digbeth Centre *(South Birmingham College)*

Edgbaston	Five Ways Island Five Ways Station, Booking Hall *(London Midland)* University Station, Booking Hall *(London Midland)* 'Nandos', 5A Five Ways Leisure Centre *(Nandos)* BowlPlex Birmingham, Broadway Plaza *(BowlPlex)* County Ground *(Warwickshire CCC)*
Erdington	Wilton Road/High Street 'Charlie Hall', Barnabas Road *(JDW)* 'Nandos', The Fort Shopping Park *(Nandos)* Gala Bingo, Streetly Road *(Gala)*
Hall Green	Hall Green Campus (2) *(South Birmingham College)*
Handsworth	Baker Street, off Soho Road
Harborne	High Street 'Old House at Home',Lordswood Road *(Private)* 'Proverbial', High Street *(Barracuda)* Gala Bingo, High Street *(Gala)*
Highgate	Gooch Street
Hockley	Vyse Street, Jewellery Quarter
Kings Heath	Vicarage Road 'Pear Tree', Alcester Road South *(JDW)*
Kings Norton	Kings Norton Station, Booking Hall *(London Midland)*
Kingstanding	Kingstanding Road
Longbridge	Longbridge Station, Booking Hall *(London Midland)*
Lozells	Boulton Road Lozells Road/Heathfield Road

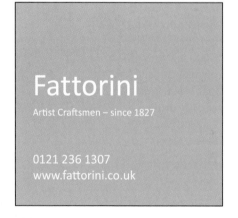
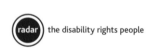
NATIONAL KEY SCHEME GUIDE 2011

Moseley		Alcester Road, by St Marys Row
		'Elizabeth of York', St Mary's Row *(JDW)*
Nechells		'Nandos', Star City *(Nandos)*
		'Old Orleans', Star City *(Private)*
Northfield		Church Road Car Park
		Northfield Station, Booking Hall *(London Midland)*
		Bournville College, Bristol Rd South *(College)*
		'Black Horse', Bristol Rd South *(JDW)*
Perry Barr		'Arthur Robertson', Walsall Road *(JDW)*
Selly Oak		Bristol Road/Harborne Lane
		Selly Oak Station, Booking Hall *(London Midland)*
Small Heath		Coventry Road/Regent Park Road
Sparkhill		Stratford Road, Sparkhill Park
Stechford		Pool Way Shopping Centre
Stirchley		Pershore Road, opp Hazlewell Street
Sutton Coldfield		Boldmere Road/Jockey Road
		The Mall Gracechurch *(Private)*
		'Bishop Vesey', Boldmere Road *(JDW)*
		'Boot Inn', Rectory Road *(Private)*
		'Bottle of Sack', Birmingham Road *(JDW)*
Walmley		Crawford Street
Weoley Castle		Weoley Castle Road
Wythall		Chapel Lane Caravan Club Site *(Caravan Club)*
Yardley		Gala Bingo, Swan Centre, Coventry Rd *(Gala)*

Bromsgrove

Alvechurch		Tanyard Lane
Bromsgrove	**CP**	Crown Close, Market Street
		Sanders Park
		'Golden Cross Hotel', High Street *(JDW)*
Frankley M5		Frankley Services, J3/4 M5 *(Moto)*
Rubery		New Road

Cannock Chase

Cannock	'Linford Arms', High Green *(JDW)*
	Green Building, Cannock Campus *(S Staffs College)*
Hendesford	Cannock Chase Visitor Centre *(Staffs CC)*
Rugeley	'The Plaza', Horsefair *(JDW)*

Coventry

Ansty	'Ansty Arms', Combe Fields Road *(Private)*
Canley	Neighbourhood Office
Cannon Park	De Montfort Way Shopping Centre
Cheylesmore	Daventry Road/Cecily Road
Coventry City Centre	Belgrade Plaza Car Park, off Hill Street
	British Road Transport Museum (Museum hrs)
	Central Library (Library hrs)
	Pool Meadow Bus Station *(Centro)*
	Cathedral Lanes Shopping Centre *(Private)*
	Lower Precinct Shopping Centre *(Private)*
	West Orchard Shopping Centre *(Private)*
	Coventry Station, Platform 1 *(Virgin)*
	'Earl of Mercia', High Street *(JDW)*
	'Flying Standard', Trinity Street *(JDW)*
	'Nandos', Trinity Street *(Nandos)*
	'Old Orleans', The Sky Dome *(Private)*
	'Spon Gate', The Skydome *(JDW)*
	'Varsity', Little Park Street *(Barracuda)*
	Belgrade Theatre *(Private)*
	Gala Bingo, Radford Road *(Gala)*
Earlsdon	Library, Albany Road
	'City Arms', Earlsdon Street *(JDW)*
Edgwick	Edgwick Park, Foleshill Road
Gosford Green	Binley Road/Walsgrave Road
Radford	Jubilee Crescent Shopping Centre
Tile Hill	Tile Hill Station *(London Midland)*
Walsgrave	'Nandos', Gielug Way *(Nandos)*

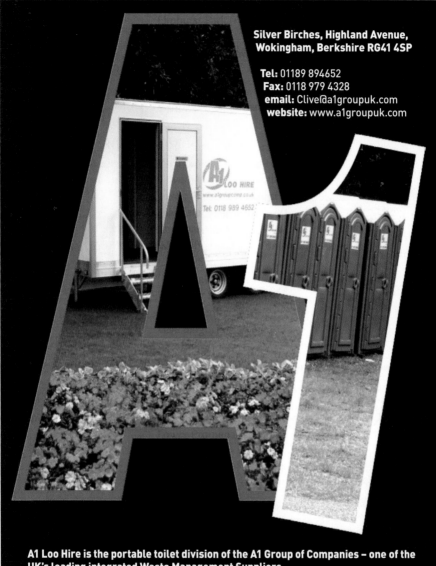

Silver Birches, Highland Avenue, Wokingham, Berkshire RG41 4SP

Tel: 01189 894652
Fax: 0118 979 4328
email: Clive@a1groupuk.com
website: www.a1groupuk.com

A1 Loo Hire is the portable toilet division of the A1 Group of Companies – one of the UK's leading integrated Waste Management Suppliers.

Our extensive range of hygienic toilets are available from our depots in Wokingham, Coventry and Bridgend, South Wales for any outdoor event or construction project.

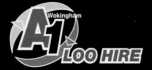

Dudley

Amblecote	Sainsbury's Store, Sandringham Way *(Sainsbury)*
Brierley Hill	Little Cottage Street 'Corn Exchange', Amblecote Road *(Private)*
Coseley	Castle Street Coseley Station, Platform 2 *(London Midland)*
Dudley	Flood Street Car Park (M+F) Market Place Bus Station, Birmingham Street *(Centro)* 'Full Moon', High Street *(JDW)* 'Nandos', Castlegate *(Nandos)* Dudley BowlPlex, Castlegaste *(BowlPlex)* Gala Bingo, Castle Hill *(Gala)*
Halesowen	Halesowen Bus Station *(Centro)* 'William Shenstone', Queensway *(JDW)*
Kingswinford	The Cross
Merry Hill	Debenhams Store, Pedmore Road *(Debenhams)* 'Abraham Darby', Merry Hill *(JDW)* 'Bar Edge', Level Street *(Private)*

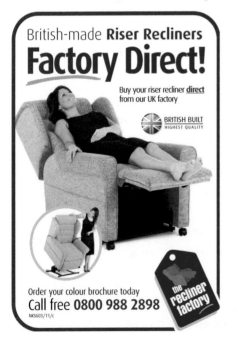
The Octagon
Shopping Centre

Is pleased to
support the
Royal Association
for Disability Rights

NATIONAL KEY SCHEME GUIDE 2011

		'Nandos', Food Court *(Nandos)*
		'Waterfront Inn', Level Street *(JDW)*
Netherton		Halesowen Road
Sedgley		Townsend Place
		'The Clifton', Bull Ring *(JDW)*
Stourbridge		Court Street, off New Road
	CP	Crystal Leisure Centre (Centre hrs)
		Ryemarket Shopping Centre *(Private)*
		Bus Station, Foster Street *(Centro)* [to reopen 2012]
		Stourbridge Junction Station, Plats. 1/2 *(London Midland)*
		'Chequers Inn', High Street *(JDW)*
		'Edward Rutland', High Street *(JDW)*
Wollaston		Meridan Avenue

East Staffordshire

Barton-under-Needwood	Crowberry Lane, off Main Street
Branston	Branston Water Park (Park hrs)
	'The Gate', Main Street *(Private)*
Burton-on-Trent	Manor Croft, Market Place
	Shobnall Leisure Complex (Centre hrs)
	Station Road
	Town Hall (Office hrs)
	Register Office & Consumer Direct (Office hrs) *(Staffs CC)*
	Octagon Shopping Centre *(Private)*
	'The Albion', Shobnall Road *(Marstons)*
	'Barracuda', Station Street *(Barracuda)*
	'Cosmopolitan Bar', High Street *(Private)*
	'Lord Burton', High Street *(JDW)*
	'Wing Wah Restaurant', New Street *(Private)*
	Mecca Bingo, Middleway Park *(Private)*
Rolleston-on-Dove	'Spread Eagle', Church Road *(M&B)*
Stapenhill	Main Street
	'Crown Inn', Rosildon Road *(Private)*
Stretton	'Mill House', Milford Drive *(Private)*
Tutbury	Duke Street Car Park
	'Dog & Partridge', High Street *(Private)*
Uttoxeter	Bradley Street
	Bramshall Road Recreation Ground

Trinity Road Car Park
'The Academy', Market Place *(Barracuda)*
'Old Swan', Market Place *(JDW)*
Uttoxeter Racecourse Caravan Club Site *(Caravan Club)*

Winshill Berry Hedge Youth Centre (Centre hrs)

Herefordshire

Hereford Mayford Orchards Shopping Centre (7.30-19.00)
CP Hereford Leisure Pool (Pool hrs)
Hereford Station *(Arriva Wales)*
'Kings Fee', Commercial Road *(JDW)*

Kington Mill Street

Ledbury Bye Street Car Park (8.00-19.00)
Church Lane (8.00-18.00)

Leominster Broad Street Car Park
Central Par Park
Grange (6.00-17.00)
CP Leominster Leisure Centre (Centre hrs)

Malvern Hills British Camp
Colwell

Moorhampton Moorhampton Caravan Club Site *(Caravan Club)*

Ross-on-Wye Croft Shopping Centre (8.00-19.00)
Wye Street
'Mail Rooms', Gloucester Road *(JDW)*

Weobley Back Lane, Library Car Park

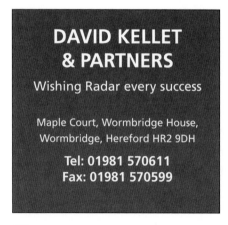
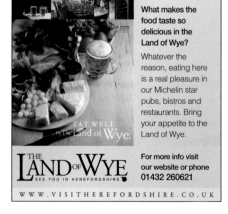

Lichfield

Burntwood	Sankeys Corner (7.30-17.30) Swan Island (9.00-17.30)
Chasetown	High Street (7.30-17.00)
Lichfield	Bus Station, Birmingham Road (7.00-18.00) Dam Street (9.00-17.30) Friary (8.00-17.30) Swan Road (9.00-17.30) 'Acorn Inn', Tamworth Street *(JDW)* 'Gatehouse', Bird Street *(JDW)*

Malvern Hills

Bransford	'Fox Inn', Bransford Court Lane *(Private)*
Great Malvern	Barnards Green (7.00-19.00) Grange Road (7.00-19.00) Great Malvern Station, Platform 1 *(London Midland)*
Hanley Swan	Blackmore Caravan Club Site *(Caravan Club)*
Malvern Link	Victoria Pavilion *(Town Council)*
Tenbury Wells	Teme Street Car Park (7.00-19.00)
Upton-upon-Severn	Hanley Road Car Park High Street

Newcastle-Under-Lyme

Kidsgrove	Heathcote Street (8.00-18.00)
Newcastle-under-Lyme	Bradwell Park

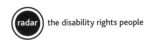 the disability rights people

Get Caravanning

A guide to helping you explore caravanning from a disabled person's point of view.

Available from Radar's online shop
www.radar-shop.org.uk

NEWCASTLE
U N D E R ▲ L Y M E
BOROUGH COUNCIL

For more information on Public Facilities and access to many attractions why not telephone for more details before you travel?

Please telephone for all enquiries:

01782 742 500

Chesterton Park
Hassell Street
Merrial Street
Westlands Sports Centre
Wolstanton Marsh
Wolstanton Park
Sainsbury's Store, Liverpool Rd *(Sainsbury)*
'Arnold Machin', Ironmarket *(JDW)*
'Yates's Bar', Ironmarket *(Yates)*

North Warwickshire

Atherstone	Bus Station
Coleshill	High Street
	Coleshill Parkway Station, Booking Hall *(London Midland)*
	'Bell Inn', Birmingham Road *(Private)*
Water Orton	Birmingham Road

Nuneaton & Bedworth

Bedworth	Civic Hall (Hall hrs)
	Chapel Street (9.00-17.30. Mon-Sat)
	Market Place (9.00-17.30. Mon-Sat)
	'Bear & Ragged Staff', King Street *(JDW)*
Nuneaton	Bus Station
	Ropewalk Shopping Centre MSCP (Centre hrs)
	Town Hall, Coton Road (Office hrs)
	Nuneaton Station, Platform 6 *(London Midland)*
	Sainsbury's Store, Vicarage St *(Sainsbury)*
	'Felix Holt', Stratford Street *(JDW)*
	'William White', Newdegate Street *(JDW)*
CP	Resource Centre, Abbey Street (Centre hrs)

Redditch

Redditch	Redditch Town Hall, Walter Stranz Sq (Office hrs)
	Threadneedle House, Alcester St (Office hrs)
	Woodrow Centre One Stop Shop (Office hrs)
	Kingfisher Shopping Centre (5) *(Private)*
	Redditch Station, Booking Hall *(London Midland)*
	'Foxlydiate', Birchfield Road *(Private)*
	'Rising Sun', Alcester Street *(JDW)*

'Royal Enfield', Unicorn Hill *(JDW)*

Rugby

Coombe Abbey	Countryside Park, Visitor Centre *(Coventry)*
Rugby	Benn Hall, Newbold Road (Hall hrs)
	Caldecott Park (Daytime)
	Ken Marriott Leisure Centre (Centre hrs)
	Newbold Quarry
	North Street Car Park
	Rugby Art Gallery, Museum & Library (2) (Building hrs)
	Visitors' Centre, Art Gallery & Museum (Centre hrs)
	Churchside Arcade *(Private)*
	Clock Towers Shopping Centre (2) *(Private)*
	Frobisher Road Pavilion *(Private)*
	Rugby Station, Platform 2 *(Virgin)*
	'Rupert Brooke', Castle Street *(JDW)*
	Gala Bingo, North Street *(Gala)*

Sandwell

Cradley Heath	Lower High Street, Car Park (9.00-17.30)
	Bus Station, Forge Lane *(Centro)*
	Cradley Heath Station, by Platform 1 *(London Midland)*
	'Moon Under Water', High Street *(JDW)*
Great Barr	Scott Arms Shopping Centre
	Gala Bingo, Walsall Road *(Gala)*
Oldbury	Sandwell & Dudley Station, Car Park
Rowley Regis	Henderson Way, Car Park

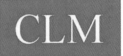

	'The Britannia', Halesowen Street *(JDW)*
Smethwick	Stoney Lane, Car Park (9.00-17.30) Bearwood Bus Station, Adkins Lane *(Centro)* 'Sampson Lloyd', Cape Hill *(JDW)*
Wednesbury	The Shambles Bus Station, Holyhead Road *(Centro)* 'The Bellwether', Walsall Street *(JDW)* Gala Bingo, St James Bridge *(Gala)*
West Bromwich	Sandwell Valley Country Park (7) Bus Station, Ring Road (6.00-24.00) *(Centro)* The Hawthorns Station, Booking Hall *(London Midland)* Sandwell Centre, Kings Square *(Private)* Sandwell Centre, Queens Square *(Private)* 'Billiard Hall', St Michael's Ringway *(JDW)*

Shropshire

Albrighton	Crown Car Park
Bishops Castle	Station Street Car Park
Bridgnorth	Fox Corner, St John's Street Innage Lane Car Park Listley Street Car Park Castle Grounds (Park hrs) *(Town Council)* Sainsbury's Store, Whitburn Street *(Sainsburys)* 'Jewel of the Severn', High Street *(JDW)*
Broseley	Dark Lane Car Park
Church Stretton	Easthope Road Car Park Carding Mill Valley *(National Trust)*
Clee Hill	High Street, A4117
Clun	Newcastle Road Car Park
Craven Arms	Shrewsbury Road
Ellesmere	Cross Street
Ford	A458 Lay-by
Gobowen	Gobowen Station *(Arriva Wales)*
Highley	High Street Car Park
Ludlow	Castle Street Car Park Smithfield Car Park

Ludlow Station *(Arriva Wales)*
British Legion Club, Mill Street *(RBL)*

Market Drayton	Towers Lawn 1 Car Park 'Hippodrome', Queen Street *(JDW)*
Much Wenlock	St Mary's Lane Car Park
Oswestry	Beatrice Street Car Park Central Car Park, English Walls *(Town Council)* Cae Glass Park *(Town Council)* 'Wilfred Owen', Willow Street *(JDW)*
Pontesbury	School Bank
Prees Heath	Car & Lorry Park
Shifnal	Aston Street Car Park
Shrewsbury	Raven Meadow Car Park (8.00-18.30) Abbey Foregate (8.00-17.00) *(Town Council)* Hills Lane (8.00-17.00) *(Town Council)* Quarry Bottom (Daytime) *(Town Council)* Quarry Top (Daytime) *(Town Council)* Sydney Avenue (8.00-16.30) *(Town Council)* Shrewsbury Station *(Arriva Wales)* 'Nandos', Old Potts Way *(Nandos)* 'Shrewsbury Hotel', Bridge Place *(JDW)* Gala Bingo, Castle Gate *(Gala)*
Snailbeach	Village Hall
Wem	High Street Car Park
Whitchurch	Brownlow Street White Lion Meadow

Solihull

Berkswell	'Bear Inn', Spencer Lane *(Private)*
Castle Bromwich	'The Farthings', Green Lane *(Private)*
Chelmsley Wood	Chelmsley Wood Library (Library hrs) Chelmsley Wood Shopping Centre *(Private)*
Dorridge	Dorridge Station, Platform 1 *(London Midland)* 'Drum & Monkey', Four Ashes Road *(Private)*
Marston Green	Marston Green Station, Booking Hall *(London Midland)* 'Marston Green Tavern', Station Road *(Private)*

NEC	Birmingham International Station *(Virgin)* 'Little Owl', Bickenhill Parkway *(M&B)*
Olton	Olton Station, Booking Hall *(London Midland)*
Sheldon	Rileys Snooker, Hobs Moat Road *(Private)*
Shirley	'Colebrook Inn', Haslucks Green Rd *(M&B)* 'The Drawbridge', Drawbridge Road *(Private)* 'Nandos', 186 Stratford Road *(Nandos)* 'Plume of Feathers', Stratford Road *(Private)* 'Sharmans Cross', Prospect Lane *(Private)* 'Woodmans Rest', Union Street *(Private)*
Solihull	Mell Square Solihull Arts Complex (Centre hrs) Solihull Central Library (Library hrs) Touchwood Shopping Centre *(Private)* Solihull Station, Platforms 1/2 *(London Midland)* 'Apres Bar', Poplar Road *(Private)* 'Assembley Rooms', Poplar Road *(JDW)* 'Boat Inn', Catherine de Barnes *(Private)* 'Coach House', Herbert Road *(Marstons)* 'Druckers Café', Touchwood Centre *(Private)* 'Greville Arms', Damson Lane *(M&B)* 'Jimmy Spices', Station Road *(Private)* 'Nandos', Mill Lane Arcade *(Nandos)* 'Nog', Station Road *(Private)* 'O'Neils', Poplar Road *(Private)* 'Saddlers Arms', Warwick Road *(Private)* 'Slug & Lettuce', Touchwood Centre *(Private)* 'Town House', Warwick Road *(Private)* 'White Swan', Station Road *(JDW)*
Widney Manor	Widney Manor Station, Booking Hall *(London Midland)*

South Staffordshire

Essington M6	Hilton Park Services, J10a/11 M6 *(Moto)*
Himley	'Himley House' *(Private)*

Stafford

Little Haywood	Jubilee Playing Fields *(Parish Council)*
Milford	Brocton Lane (M+F)
Stafford	Bridge Street MSCP, opp Civic Centre
	Broad Street Car Park, by Shopmobility
	Civic Centre, Ground Floor (Office hrs)
	Doxey Road Lorry Park
	North Walls Car Park
	Rowley Park Sports Stadium (Park hrs)
	Stafford Castle Visitor Centre, Newport Road
	Stafford Crematorium (8.00-dusk)
	Stafford Market (M+F) (Market hrs)
	Victoria Park (Park hrs)
	Stafford Station, Platform 1 *(Virgin)*
	'Picture House', Bridge Street *(JDW)*
	Gala Bingo, Silkmore Lane *(Gala)*
Stone	Crown Street Car Park
	Station Road
	'Post of Stone', Granville Square *(JDW)*
Stone M6	Stafford North Services, J14/15 M6 *(Moto)*

Staffordshire Moorlands

Alstonfield	Car Park *(Peak District NP)*
Biddulph	Biddulph Grange Country Park
	Town Hall
	Wharf Road Car Park
	Greenway Bank Country Park *(Staffs CC)*
	'Bradley Green', High Street *(JDW)*
Blythe Bridge	Cheadle Road
Cheadle	Tape Street Car Park
Cheddleton	Deep Hayes Country Park *(Staffs CC)*
Cotton	The Star Caravan & Camping Park *(Private)*
Hulme End	Visitor Centre (Centre hrs)
Ilam	Wetton Mill, Ilam Park *(National Trust)*
Leek	Bus Station, Smithfield Centre
	Silk Street Car Park (7.00-18.00)

	Blackshaw Moor Caravan Club Site *(Caravan Club)*
Mildale	Mildale Village
Oakamoor	Oakamoor Picnic Areas *(Staffs CC)*
Rudyard	Lakeside (Visitor Centre hrs)
Waterhouses	Car Park *(Peak District NP)*
Wetley Rocks	Consall Nature Park *(Staffs CC)*
Wetton	Wetton Village

Stoke-On-Trent

Abbey Hulton	Abbey Hulton Local Centre, Abbots Rd (Office hrs)
Blurton	Blurton Local Centre, Finstock Ave (Office hrs) 'Gables', Trentham Road *(Marstons)*
Chell Heath	Chell Heath Local Centre, Cornhill Rd (Office hrs)
Etruria	Odeon Cinema, Festival Park *(Odeon)* Tenpin, Marina Way *(Private)*
Fenton	City Road Car Park, Fenton Markwet 'KFC', King Street *(KFC)* Gala Bingo, Victoria Road *(Gala)*
Hanley	Crown Bank, Stafford Street Dudson Centre, Hope Street (Centre hrs) Hanley Park, Shelton
	CP Potteries Shopping Centre *(Private)*
	Debenhams Store, Potteries Centre *(Debenhams)*
	'Caffe Nero', Parliament Road *(Private)*
	'Reginald Mitchell', Parliament Row *(JDW)*
	'Varsity', Percy Street *(Barracuda)*
	'Walkabout', Trinity Street *(Private)*
	Dudson Museum, Hope Street *(Private)*
	Gala Bingo, Albion Square *(Gala)*
	Grosvenor Casino, The Octagon *(Private)*
Longton	Longton Local Centre, Commerce St (Office hrs) Longton Market, Transport St. (Market hrs)
Meir	Meir Local Centre, Uttoxeter Rd (Office hrs) Weston Road Car Park
Milton	Carmontside Cemetery (Cemetery hrs)
Norton	Norton Local Centre, St Nicholas Ave (Office hrs)

Packmoor	'Brindley's Lock', Silverstone Crescent *(Private)*
Smallthorne	Community Drive
Stoke	Kingsway Car Park South Wolfe Street Market Stoke-on-Trent Station *(Virgin)* 'The Wheatsheaf', Church Street *(JDW)*
Trent Vale	Michelin Athletics Club, Rosetree Ave *(Private)*
Tunstall	Butterfield Place (2) Tunstall Park
Weston Coyney	Park Hall Country Park (2)

Stratford On Avon

Alcester	Bulls Head Yard, Car Park 'Royal Oak', High Street *(Private)*
Bidford-on-Avon	High Street Big Meadow *(Parish Council)*
Earlswood	'Reservoir', The Common *(Private)*
Henley-in-Arden	Station Road

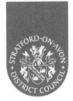

Public Conveniences

Eleven sites throughout the district
with Radar key facilities. For
information/locations
Call 01789 267 575

Stratford Shopmobility

Open on six days, based in
Stratford-upon-Avon

Call 01789 414 534

Shipston-on-Stour	Telegraph Street
Southam	Wood Street
Stratford-upon-Avon	Avonbank Gardens, Old Town
	Bridgefoot, Car Park
	Recreation Ground, Play Area
	Waterside (M+F)
	Windsor Street, Car Park
	Town Square Shopping Centre *(Private)*
	Visitor & Leisure Centre, Bridgeway *(Private)*
	'Golden Bee', Sheep Street *(JDW)*
	'Ripple Café', Swans Nest Lane *(Private)*
Studley	Birmingham Road
Warmington	'Wobbly Wheel', Warwick Road *(Private)*

Tamworth

Tamworth	Aldergate (8.00-6.00)
	Castle Pleasure Grounds (Park hrs)
	Wiggington Road Cemetery (Cemetery hrs)
	Ankerside Shopping Centre *(Private)*
	Co-op Store, Colehill *(Private)*
	'The Bolebridge', Bolebridge Street *(JDW)*
	'Silk Kite', Church Street *(JDW)*
	'Yates's Bar', Lower Gungate *(Yates)*
Tamworth, M42	Tamworth Services, J10 M42/A5 *(Moto)*

Telford & Wrekin

Brookside		Brookside Community Centre
Dawley		King Street *(Parish Council)*
Hadley		District Centre *(Parish Council)*
Ironbridge		The Square
		The Wharfage
	CP	Self Unlimited *(Private)*
Madeley		High Street *(Parish Council)*
Malinslee		Town Park *(Parish Council)*
Newport		Stafford Street Car Park *(Town Council)*
Oakengates		Stafford Road *(Parish Council)*

Sutton Hill	Sutton Hill Community Centre
Telford	Telford Shopmobility, Red Oak Car Park *(Private)*
	Telford Shopping Centre (3) *(Private)*
	Debenhams Store, Sherwood Sq *(Debenhams)*
	Telford Centre Bus Station *(Private)*
	Telford Central Station, Booking Hall *(London Midland)*
	'Thomas Botfield', Telford Shopping Centre *(JDW)*
	SA Building, Telford Campus *(Univ of Wolverhampton)*
	Student Union, Telford Campus *(Univ of Wolverhampton)*
Wellington	The Parade *(Town Council)*
	Walker Street *(Town Council)*

Walsall

Aldridge	Anchor Road, Shopping Precinct
	Gala Bingo, Anchor Road *(Gala)*
Blakenall	Blakenall Shopping Centre
Bloxwich	High Street/Wolverhampton Road
	Asda, High Street
Pelsall	Norton Road
Walsall	St Pauls Bus Station (7.00-21.00) *(Centro)*
	Walsall Station, Booking Hall *(London Midland)*
	'The Imperial', Darwall Street *(JDW)*
	'Park Tavern', Broadway North *(Private)*
	'Varsity', Darwall Street *(Barracuda)*
	'Yates's Bar', Leicester Street *(Yates)*
	WC Building, Walsall Campus *(Univ of Wolverhampton)*
	Gala Bingo, Jerome Retail Park *(Gala)*
Willenhall	Market Car Park
	'The Malthouse', New Road *(JDW)*

Warwick

Kenilworth	Abbey End (Daytime)
	Abbey Fields (Daytime)
	Kenilworth Cemetery (Cemetery hrs)
Lapworth	Brome Hall Lane (Summer) *(Parish Council)*
Leamington Spa	Brunswick Street (Daytime)
	Covent Gardens MSCP (Daytime)
	Jephson Gardens (Daytime)

	Leamington Cemetery (Daytime) Regent Grove (Daytime) Leamington Spa Station, Platform 2 *(Chiltern Rlwy)* 'Benjamin Satchwell', The Parade *(JDW)*
Lillington	Crown Way (Daytime)
Radford Semele	'White Lion', Southam Road *(Private)*
Warwick	Market Place (Daytime) Myton Fields (Summer and weekends, daytime) Pageant Gardens (Daytime) St Nicholas Park (Daytime) Warwick Cemetery (Cemetery hrs) **CP** Shire Hall *(Warwicks CC)* 'Thomas Lloyd', Market Place *(JDW)* 'Varsity', Gibbett Hill Road *(Barracuda)* Warwick Racecourse Caravan Club Site *(Caravan Club)*

Wolverhampton

Bilston	Market (7.00-21.00) Bus Station *(Centro)* [to reopen mid-2011] Bilston Craft Gallery *(Private)* 'Sir Henry Newbold', High Street *(JDW)*
Compton	'Odd Fellows', Compton Road *(Marstons)*
Merry Hill	'Merry Hill', Trysull Road *(Private)*
Tettenhall	Stockwell Road (7.00-21.00)
Wednesfield	High Street (7.00-21.00) 'Royal Tiger', High Street *(JDW)*

AMF Bowl Bentley Bridge *(AMF)*

Wolverhampton Art Gallery, Lichfield Street (Gallery hrs)
Ashmore Park, Griffiths Drive (7.00-18.00)
Civic Centre, St Peters Square
Faulkland Street Coach Station (7.00-19.00)
WCityStop, Mander Centre (Mon-Sat, 9.00-17.00)
Wolverhampton Market, School Street
West Park (Park hrs)
Bus Station, Pipers Row *(Centro)*
Mander Shopping Centre *(Private)*
Wulfrun Shopping Centre (2) *(Private)*
Beatties Store, Victoria Street *(Private)*
Littlewoods Store, Bilston Street *(Private)*
Wolverhampton Station, Platform 1 *(Virgin)*
Bantock House Café, Finchfield Rd *(Private)*
'Edwards', North Street *(M&B)*
'Goose in the City', Lichfield Street *(M&B)*
'Hog's Head', Stafford Street *(Private)*
'Moon Under Water', Lichfield Street *(JDW)*
'Nandos', 23 Queen Street *(Nandos)*
'Oceana', Bilston Street *(Private)*
'O'Neills', Lichfield Street *(M&B)*
'Revolution', Princess Street *(Private)*
'Rothwells', Lichfield Street *(Private)*
'Scream', Wulfruna Street *(Private)*
'The Tube', Princes Street *(Private)*
'Varsity', Stafford Street *(Barracuda)*
'Walkabout', Queen Street *(Private)*
'Yates's Bar', Queens Square *(Yates)*
CA Building, Compton Park Campus *(Wolverhampton Univ)*
MA Building, City Campus S. *(Wolverhampton Univ)*
MD Building, Students Union *(Wolverhampton Univ)*
ML Building, City Campus N. *(Wolverhampton Univ)*
Gala Bingo, Bushbury Lane *(Gala)*
Molineux Stadium *(Wolves FC)*

Worcester

Worcester Barbourne Lane (8.15-17.30)
Bull Ring, St Johns
Reindeer Court Shopping Centre *(Private)*
Shrub Hill Station. Platform 1a *(London Midland)*

'The Crown', Crown Passage *(JDW)*
'Nandos', 55 Friar Street *(Nandos)*
'Postal Order', Foregate Street *(JDW)*
Gala Bingo, Foregate Street *(Gala)*

Wychavon

Broadway	Church Close Car Park
	Milestone Ground Car Park
	Broadway Caravan Club Site *(Caravan Club)*
Droitwich	Lido Park (8.00-18.00)
	St Andrews Square
Evesham	Abbey Park (Daytime)
	Oat Street (Daytime)
	Old Brewery Car Park (9.00-18.00)
	Viaduct Meadow (Daytime)
	Waterside
	Evesham Station *(Gt Western)*
	'Old Swanne Inn', High Street *(JDW)*
Pershore	Church Walk (8.00-18.00)
	High Street Car Park (Daytime)

Wyre Forest

Bewdley	Car Park, off Load Street
	Dog Lane Car Park
	'George Hotel', Load Street *(JDW)*
	'Running Horse Inn', Long Bank *(Private)*
Kidderminster	Brintons Park, Sutton Road
	Broadwaters Park, Stourbridge Road
	Market Street (Daytime)
	Rowlands Hill Shopping Centre (7.00-17.30)
	Swan Shopping Centre *(Private)*
	Wyre Forest Glades Arena *(Private)*
	'The Penny Black', Bull Ring *(JDW)*
	'Watermill', Park Lane *(Private)*
CP	Connect, Blackwell Street *(Worcs CC)*
Lower Arley	Frenchman Street
Stourport-on-Severn	Raven Street Car Park
	Severn Meadows Car Park, by Civic Centre
	Vale Road Car Park
	'Ye Olde Crown', Bridge Street *(JDW)*

NORTH WEST ENGLAND

Allerdale

Allonby	Central Green, by Play Area
	West Green
Aspatria	Queen Street Car Park
Buttermere	Village Car Park *(Lake District NP)*
Cockermouth	Harris Park (Daytime)
	Main Street (Daytime)
Keswick	Belle Close Car Park
	Central Car Park
	Lakeside Car Park, behind Theatre
	Station Platform
Maryport	Harbour, Irish Street
	High Street
Rosthwaite	By Car Park *(Lake District NP)*
Silloth	The Green
	Skinburness, opp. Solway Village
Wigton	Market Hall (Daytime)
Workington	Harrington Marina
	Town Centre (Daytime)
	'Henry Bessemer', New Oxford Street *(JDW)*

Barrow-In-Furness

Barrow-in-Furness	Amphitheatre, Manor Road
	Barrow Park, The Pavilion (Park hrs)
	Fell Street, Car Park
	Roa Island
	Debenhams Store, Portland Wk *(Debenhams)*
	'The Furness Railway', Abbey Road *(JDW)*
	'Yates's Bar', Duke Street *(Yates)*
Dalton-in-Furness	Tudor Square
Walney Island	Earnse Bay, Westshore Road

Blackburn With Darwen

Blackburn	Market Way

Witton Country Park, Preston Old Road
The Mall Blackburn (2) *(Private)*
Debenhams Store, Northgate *(Debenhams)*
Blackburn Station *(Northern Rail)*
'Boddington Arms', Myerscough Road *(Private)*
'The Postal Order', Darwen Street *(JDW)*
Blackburn College (7) *(College)*
BowlPlex, Peel Leisure Park *(BowlPlex)*
Gala Bingo, Ainsworth Street *(Gala)*

Darwen	Town Hall, Parliament Street
Roddlesworth	Ryal Fold Information Centre *(Utd Utilities)*

Blackpool

Blackpool – Central	Bethesda Square, Central Drive
	Blackpool Council Offices (Office hrs)
	Carleton Cremetorium
	Central Car Park, Central Drive/New Bonny Rd
	Layton Square, Westcliffe Drive
	Lonsdale Coach Park
	Lytham Road/Station Road

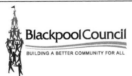

Blackpool Council
BUILDING A BETTER COMMUNITY FOR ALL

New fully modernised facilities are available throughout Blackpool. All providing a 24 hour service. Each location is accessible with a RADAR key and has baby changing facilities

Our toilets can be found at:

Little Bispham (p)	Victoria Street
Cabin (p)	Bethesda Square
Bispham Village (p)	Lonsdale Coach Park
Layton Square (p)	Lytham Road
Gynn Square (p)	Highfield Road
Cocker Square	Harrowside
Central Car Park	Starr Gate (p)
	Bispham Tram Station (p)

(p) = Located on the Promenade
All locations have facilities for the disabled
Visit our website www.blackpool.gov.uk and view the location map

	Talbot Road Bus Station
	Town Hall, Talbot Square (Office hrs)
	Victoria Street, Town Centre
	Magistrates Court *(Courts Service)*
	Festival Shopping Mall *(Private)*
	Blackpool North Station *(Northern Rail)*
	Blackpool Pleasure Beach (3) *(Private)*
CP	Blackpool Tower *(Private)*
	Central Pier, Family Bar *(Private)*
	North Pier *(Private)*
	South Pier Amusements *(Private)*
	Winter Gardens *(Private)*
	'Albert & The Lion', Bank Hey Street *(JDW)*
	'The Auctioneer', Lytham Road *(JDW)*
	'Belle Vue', Whitegate Drive *(Private)*
	'Brannigans', Market Street *(Private)*
	'King Edward VII Hotel', Central Drive *(Private)*
	'Litten Tree', Queen Street *(Private)*
	'Outside Inn', Whitehills Industrial Pk *(Private)*
	'Swift Hound', Festival Park *(Private)*
	'Walkabout', Queen Street *(Private)*
	'Yates's Bar', 407-411 The Promenade *(Yates)*
CP	Centre for Independent Living (Centre hrs)

Blackpool – North	Bispham Tram Station, Queens Promenade
	Bispham Village Car Park
	Cocker Square/Promenade
	Gynn Square, Promenade
	Little Bispham, Queens Prom/Princes Way
	Uncle Tom's Cabin, Queens Promenade
	'The Highlands', 206 Queens Promenade *(Private)*
	'Red Lion', Devonshire Sq., Bispham *(Private)*
	Thornton Building, Bispham Site *(Blackpool & Fylde Coll.)*

Blackpool – South	Central Gateway
	Harrowside, Promenade South
	Highfield Road, by Library
	Starr Gate Tram Loop
CP	Solaris Centre, New South Promenade (Centre hrs)

| **Marton** | 'Clifton Arms', Preston New Road *(Private)* |
| | Blackpool South Caravan Club Site *(Caravan Club)* |

Bolton

Bolton	Moor Lane Bus Station
	Old Hall Street (Mon-Sat, 8.30-17.30)
CP	Topp Way MSCP
	Compton Place, Car Park *(Private)*
	Bolton Station, nr Footbridge *(Northern Rail)*
	Jumbles Country Park *(Utd Utilities)*
	'Nandos', Middlebrook Retail Park *(Nandos)*
	'Spinning Mule', Nelson Square *(JDW)*
	'Varsity', Churchgate *(Barracuda)*
	'Yates's Bar', Bradshawgate *(Yates)*
Farnworth	Farnworth Bus Station [Closed at present]
	Moses Gate Country Park
Horwich	Captain Street
	Horwich Parkway Station *(Northern Rail)*
	Hollywood Bowl, Middlebrook Leisure Park *(AMF)*
Westhoughton	Market Street
	'Robert Shaw', Market Street *(JDW)*

Burnley

Burnley	Briarcliffe Road, by Hospital
	Burnley Bus Station (5.00-23.30)
	Cemetery Chapel, Rossendale Road (Chapel hrs)
	Market Hall (Trading hrs)
	Millennium Car Park, Brick Street (8.00-18.00)
	Queens Park (Park hrs)
	Scott Park (Park hrs)

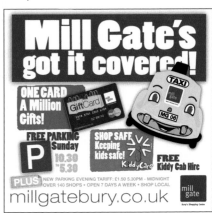

	Thompson Park, Ormerod Road (Park hrs)
	Yorkshire Street
	Burnley Central Station *(Northern Rail)*
	'Brun Lea', Manchester Road *(JDW)*
	'Walkabout', Hammerton Street *(Private)*
	Gala Bingo Club, Centenary Way *(Gala)*
Padiham	Church Street

Bury

Bury	Bus Interchange
	Kay Gardens
	Mill Gate Shopping Centre *(Private)*
	'Art Picture House', Haymarket Street *(JDW)*
	'Nandos', The Rock, Rochdale Rd *(Nandos)*
	'Robert Peel', Market Place *(JDW)*
	'Yates's Bar', Market Street *(Yates)*
	AMF Bowling, Rock Place *(AMF)*
	Burrs Country Park Caravan Club Site *(Caravan Club)*
CP	The Met, Market Street (Centre hrs)
Prestwich	Longfield Precinct
Radcliffe	Market Hall
Ramsbottom	Market Chambers
Tottington	Market Street

Carlisle

Brampton	Milburn Court (Daytime)
	Talkin Tarn (Park hrs)
Carlisle	Bitts Park (Park hrs)
	Covered Market (Trading hrs)
	Old Town Hall, English Street
	St Nicholas Bridge
	Town Dyke Orchard Car Park (Daytime)
	Upperby Park (Daytime)
	Debenhams Store. The Lanes *(Debenhams)*
	The Lanes Shopping Centre *(Private)*
	Carlisle Station, Platforms 1 & 4 *(Virgin)*
	'Bar Code', Botchergate *(Private)*
	'Bar Suede', The Cresent *(Private)*
	'Club XS', West Walls *(Private)*

'Gosling Bridge Inn', Kingstown Road *(Private)*
'The Griffin', Court Square *(Private)*
'The Holme', Denton Street *(Private)*
'Jumpin Jaks', English Gate Plaza *(Private)*
'Leonardo's', Lonsdale Street *(Private)*
'Litten Tree', Botchergate *(Private)*
'Lloyds Bar', Botchergate *(JDW)*
'Mood', Botchergate *(Private)*
'Teza', English Gate Plaza *(Private)*
'Turf Tavern', Newmarket Road, The Sands *(Private)*
'Walkabout', English Gate Plaza *(Private)*
'William Rufus', Botchergate *(JDW)*
'Woodrow Wilson', Botchergate *(JDW)*
Carlisle Bowl, Currock Road *(AMF)*
Gala Bingo Club, Englishgate Plaza *(Gala)*

Dalston	The Square (Daytime)
Longtown	Bank Street (Daytime)
Penton	Nicolforest Public Hall (external access)
Southwaite M6	Southwaite Services, J41/42 M6 *(Moto)*
Stapleton	Stapleton Public Hall (external access)

Cheshire East

Alderley Edge	West Street The Wizard Car Park *(National Trust)* 'De Trafford', Congleton Road *(Private)*
Alsager	Crewe Road
Audlem	Cheshire Street Car Park
Bollington	Aldington Road (9.00-16.30) Poll Bank Car Park
Brereton Heath	Country Park
Congleton	Bridestones Shopping Centre Congleton Park Market Street West Heath Shopping Centre 'The Counting House', Swan Bank *(JDW)*
Crewe	Bus Station, Delamere Street Pedley Street

	Queens Park, Victoria Avenue (Park hrs) Crewe Station, Platforms 5 and 6-11 *(Virgin)* 'The Earl', Nantwich Road *(Private)* 'Gaffers Row', Victoria Street *(JDW)*
Disley	Station Approach
Handforth	Church Road 'Millers', Wilmslow Road *(Private)*
Knutsford	King Street Car Park Northwich Road Stanley Road, by Supermarket
Knutsford M6	Knutsford Services, J18/19 M6 *(Moto)*
Langley	Trentabank Car Park *(Peak Dist NP)*
Lower Peover	'Bells of Peover' The Cobbles *(Private)*
Macclesfield	Churchill Way (8.15-17.15) Park Green Riverside Park, off Beech Lane (8.45-16.15) 'Society Rooms', Park Green *(JDW)* Macclesfield Bowl, Lyme Green Bus. Park *(AMF)*
Mere	'Kilton Inn', Hoo Green *(Private)*
Middlewich	France Hayhurst Pavilion (Park hrs) Southway, off Wheelock Street Town Bridge, Leadsmithy Street
Nantwich	Civic Hall Car Park, Beam Street **CP** Nantwich Market Snowhill Car Park, Wall Lane
Poynton	Fountain Place Nelson Pit Visitor Centre (Centre hrs)
Prestbury	Bridge Green
Sandbach	High Street, by Town Hall
Timbersbrook	Pool Bank Car Park
Wilmslow	South Drive Twinnies Bridge Country Park (Weekend, daytime) 'Bollin Fee', Swan Street *(JDW)*

Cheshire West & Chester

Alvanley		'White Lion Inn', Manley Road (Private)
Barnton		Lydyett Lane (Daytime)
Cheshire Oaks		McArthur Glen Designer Outlet *(Private)*
		'Nandos', Stanney Lane *(Nandos)*
Chester		Foregate Street
	CP	Frodsham Street Car Park
		The Groves, nr Suspension Bridge (8.00-20.00)
		Little Roodee, Car/Coach Park (9.30-17.00)
		Princess Street Bus Station
		Princess Street, under Market (8.00-18.00)
		Union Street, by Grosvenor Park (Easter-Sept)
		Bus Station *(Private)*
		The Mall Grosvenor *(Private)*
		Chester Station, Concourse *(Arriva Wales)*
		'Forest House', Love Street *(JDW)*
		'Square Bottle', Foregate Street *(JDW)*
Cuddington		Norley Road (Daytime)
Dunham Hill		'Wheatsheaf', Dunham Hill *(Private)*
Ellesmere Port		Council Offices, Civic Way (Office hrs)
		Market (Market hrs)
		Town Centre (M+F) (Daytime)
		'Grace Arms', Stanney Lane *(Private)*
		'Thomas Telford', Whitby Road *(JDW)*
		'Wheatsheaf', Overpool Road *(JDW)*

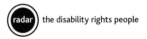 the disability rights people

Doing Work Differently

Part of our 'Doing Life Differently' series, this toolkit explores practical solutions to real questions related to work.

Available from Radar's online shop
www.radar-shop.org.uk

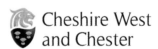 Cheshire West and Chester

Cheshire West and Chester Council support the Radar National Key Scheme

This involves the creation of a new "Changing Places" toilet at the Frodsham Street facilities opening in April 2011.

To find out more about our facilities call the council on **0300 123 8123** or email us at: **enquiries@cheshirewestandchester.gov.uk**

www. cheshirewestandchester.gov.uk

Frodsham	Moors Lane (Daytime)
Little Stanney	Chester Fairoaks Caravan Club Site *(Caravan Club)*
Neston	Brook Street
Northwich	Applemarket Street (Daytime)
	Leicester Street (Daytime)
	'Penny Black', Witton Street *(JDW)*
Parkgate	Moston Square, School Lane
Tarporley	High Street (Daytime)
Upton	Chester Zoo, The Ark Restaurant *(Private)*
Weaverham	Church Road (Daytime)
Winsford	Fountain Court [Closed at present]
	'Queens Arms', Dene Drive *(JDW)*

Chorley

Adlington	Babylon Lane
Chorley	Astley Park, Coach House
	Market Place, Cleveland Street
	Pall Mall
	'Millers', Bolton Road *(Private)*
	'Sir Henry Tate', New Market Street *(JDW)*
	Gala Bingo Club, Market Street *(Gala)*
Rivington	Great House Inf. Centre *(Utd Utilities)*
	Rivington Lane Car Park *(Utd Utilities)*
Whittle-le-Woods	'Malthouse Farm', Moss Lane *(Private)*

Copeland

Bootle	Village Car Park *(Parish Council)*
Cleator Moor	Market Place Car Park
Egremont	Chapel Street
Eskdale	The Green Station *(R&E Rlwy)*
	Ireton Road Station *(R&E Rlwy)*
Gosforth	Car Park *(Parish Council)*
Haverigg	Foreshore *(Town Council)*
Millom	The Park, St Georges Road
	Lancashire Road *(Town Council)*

Seascale	Foreshore, by Car Park
St Bees Beach	Foreshore Car Park
Whitehaven	James Street
	Whitehaven Station *(Northern Rail)*
	'Bransty Arch', Bransty Row *(JDW)*

Eden

Alston	Town Hall
	Station Car Park *(S Tynedale Rlwy)*
Appleby	Broad Close Car Park
	Tourist Information Centre, Moot Hall
Brough	Main Street
Dufton	Car Park
Garrigill	Village Hall *(Hall Committee)*
Glenridding	Jenkins Field Car Park
	Ullswater Information Centre *(Lake District NP)*
Kirkby Stephen	Stoneshot Car Park
Patterdale	opp. White Lion

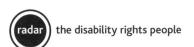
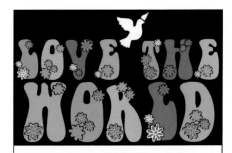

Penrith	Bluebell Lane, Little Dockray
	Castle Park
	Sandgate Bus Station/Car Park
	Penrith Station, Platform 1 *(Virgin)*
Pooley Bridge	by Tourist Information Centre
Threkeld	behind Village Hall
Troutbeck	Troutbeck Head Caravan Club Site *(Caravan Club)*

Fylde

Fairhaven Lake	Marine Park
	Stanner Bank
Freckleton	Freckleton Centre
Greenhalgh	'Fairfield Arms', Fleetwood Road *(Private)*
Kirkham	Church Street
	Kirkham & Wesham Station *(Northern Rail)*
Lytham	East Beach
	Lowther Pavilion, West Beach
	Pleasant Street Car Park
St Anne's	Fairhaven Road
	Promenade Gardens, by Monument
	St Annes Road West, by Station
	'Trawl Boat Inn', Wood Street *(JDW)*

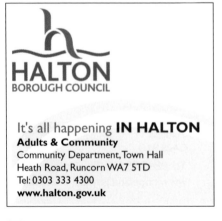
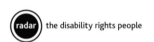
NATIONAL KEY SCHEME GUIDE 2011

Halton

Daresbury	'Ring O'Bells', Chester Road *(Private)*
Runcorn	Runcorn Station, Platform 1 *(Virgin)*
	'Ferry Boat', Church Street *(JDW)*
Widnes	'The Premier', Albert Road *(JDW)*

Hyndburn

Accrington	Peel Street Bus Station
	Arndale Shopping Centre *(Private)*
Clayton-le-Moors	Public Library
Great Harwood	Blackburn Road, Town Centre

Knowsley

Halewood	**CP**	Halewood One Stop Shop (Office hrs)
Huyton	**CP**	Municipal Buildings (Office hrs)
		Bus Station *(Merseytravel)*
Kirkby		Cherryfield Drive Bus Station
		Kirkby Market
		'Gold Balance', New Town Gardens *(JDW)*
		Gala Bingo, Telegraph Way *(Gala)*
Prescot		'Grapes Hotel', St Helens Road *(Private)*

Lancaster

Bolton-le-Sands	Community Centre *(Private)*
Carnforth	Market Square
Carnforth M6	Burton-in-Kendal Services, M6 J35/35 *(Moto)*
Caton	Bull Beck Picnic Area
	Crook of Lune Car Park *(Lancs CC)*
Glasson Dock	Condor Green Picnic Area *(Lancs CC)*
Heysham	Village Car Park *(Parish Council)*
Lancaster	Williamson Park (Park hrs)
	Bus Station *(Private)*
	Nelson Street Car Park *(Private)*
	Marketgate *(Private)*
	Market Hall *(Private)*
	St Nicholas Arcade *(Private)*

	Lancaster Station Platforms 3 & 4 *(Virgin)*
	Alexander Square *(Lancaster University)*
	'Green Ayre', North Road *(JDW)*
	'Sir Richard Owen', Spring Garden St *(JDW)*
	'Varsity', George Street *(Barracuda)*
	Lancaster & Morecambe College, A Block *(College)*
	Gala Bingo Club, King Street *(Gala)*
Lancaster M6	Lancaster Services, J32/33 M6 *(Moto)*
Middleton	Parish Hall *(Private)*
Morecambe	Festival Market Hall
	Happy Mount Car Park
	Library Car Park
	Promenade, Clock Tower
	Promenade, West End Gardens
	Stone Jetty *(Private)*
	'Eric Bartholomew', Euston Road *(JDW)*
	Gala Bingo Club, Marine Road East *(Gala)*
Silverdale	Gaskell Hall *(Private)*

Liverpool

Allerton	'Yates's Bar', Allerton Road *(Yates)*
Childwall	'Childwall Fiveways', Queens Drive *(JDW)*
Clark Gardens	'Allerton Hall', Springwood Avenue *(Private)*
Croxteth	Gala Bingo, Stonedale Retail Park *(Gala)*
Hunts Cross	Hunts Cross Station, Platform 3 *(MerseyRail)*
Garston	Garston Library (Library hrs)
Gateacre	'Bear & Staff', Gateacre Brow *(Private)*
Liverpool City Centre	Central Library, William Brown St (Library hrs)
	Albert Dock, Britannia Pavilion *(Private)*
	Clayton Square Shopping Centre *(Private)*
CP	Liverpool One, Wall Street *(Private)*
	St Johns Shopping Centre *(Private)*
	Coach Station, Norton St *(Nat Express)*
	Queen Square Bus Station *(Merseytravel)*
	Lime Street Station, Concourse *(Network Rail)*
	Liverpool Central Station *(MerseyRail)*
	Haigh Building, Maryland Street *(LJM University)*

Royal Liverpool Hospital *(Hospital)*
'Fall Well', St John's Way *(JDW)*
'Fly in the Loaf', Hardman Street *(Private)*
'Ha! Ha! Bar', Albert Dock *(Private)*
'Knotty Ash Hotel', East Prescot Rd *(Private)*
'Lime Kiln', Fleet Street *(JDW)*
'Nandos', Liverpool One *(Nandos)*
'Nandos', 6 Queen Square *(Nandos)*
'Norwegian Blue', Bold Street *(Private)*
'The Picturedrome', 286 Kensington *(JDW)*
'Rat & Parrot', Queen Square *(Private)*
'The Raven', Walton Vale *(JDW)*
'Richard John Blackler' , Charlotte Row *(JDW)*
'Thomas Frost', Walton Road *(JDW)*
'Wagamama', P10, Liverpool One *(Private)*
'Walkabout', Fleet Street *(Private)*
'The Welkin', Whitechapel *(JDW)*
'Yates's Bar', Queens Square *(Yates)*

Norris Green	Lifestyles Ellergate (Centre hrs)
Speke	Pizza Hut, New Mersey Retail Park *(Private)* 'The Argosy', John Lennon Airport *(JDW)*
Stoneycroft	'The Navigator', Queens Drive *(JDW)*
Toxteth	Lifestyles Toxteth (Centre hrs)
Walton	Lifestyles Alsop (Centre hrs)
Wavertree	Wavertree Technology Park Station *(Northern Rail)* Gala Bingo, Wavertree Road *(Gala)* Liverpool Aquatics Centre (Centre hrs)

Manchester

Belle Vue	Gala Bingo, Hyde Road *(Gala)*
Cheetham Hill	Humphrey Street
Chorlton-cum-Hardy	Bus Terminus, Barlow Moor Road Manchester Road 'Sedge Lynn', Manchester Road *(JDW)*
Didsbury	Barlow Moor Road, by Library 'Milson Rhodes', School Lane *(JDW)* 'Nandos', Parrs Wood Leisure *(Nandos)*
Fallowfield	'Great Central', Wilmslow Road *(JDW)*

	'Nandos', 351 Wimslow Road *(Nandos)*
Harpurhey	Gala Bingo, North City Shopping Centre *(Gala)*
Heaton Park	Sainsbury's Store, Heaton Park Rd West *(Sainsbury)*
Levenshulme	Albert Road, off Stockport Road
Manchester Airport	Bus Station *(GMPTE)*
	Manchester Airport Station *(Transpennine)*
Manchester City Centre	Castlefield, off Liverpool Street
	Church Street/Tib Street
	John Dalton Street/Deansgate
	Parker Street, Piccadilly Bus Station
	Stevenson Square
	Town Hall Extension, Mount Street (Daytime)
	Arndale Centre *(Private)*
	Shudehill Interchange *(GMPTE)*
	Deansgate Station *(Northern Rail)*
	Piccadilly Station (2) *(Network Rail)*
	Victoria Station *(Northern Rail)*
	Debenhams Store, Market St *(Debenhams)*
	'Ha! Ha! Bar', Spinningfields *(Private)*
	'Manchester & County', Piccadilly *(JDW)*
	'Moon Under Water', Deansgate *(JDW)*
	'Nandos', Arndale Centre *(Nandos)*
	'Nandos', Hardman St, Spinningfields *(Nandos)*
	'Nandos', Oxford Road *(Nandos)*
	'Nandos', The Printworks *(Nandos)*
	'Norwegian Blue', Corporation Street *(Private)*
	'Old Orleans', Withy Grove *(Private)*
	'The Paramount', Oxford Road *(JDW)*
	'Sawyers Arms', Deansgate *(Private)*
	'Seven Stars', Dantzic Street *(JDW)*
	'Varsity', The Circus, Oxford Street *(Barracuda)*
	'Varsity', Wimslow Park *(Barracuda)*
	'Walkabout', Quay Street *(Private)*
	'Waterhouse', Princess Street *(JDW)*
	'Yates's Bar', Portland Street *(Yates)*
Rusholme	'Ford Maddox Ford', Wilmslow Park *(JDW)*
Sportcity	City of Manchester Stadium *(Manchester City FC)*
Withington	Burton Road, by White Lion
	Mill Lane, off Palatine Road

Wythenshawe	Civic Centre
	Hollyhedge Road, nr. Brownley Road
	Wythenshawe Bus Station
	Gala Bingo, Rowlandsway *(Gala)*

Oldham

Chadderton	Shopping Precinct (Daytime)
Greenfield	Dovestones Reservoir
	Greenfield Station *(Northern Rail)*
Oldham	Alexandra Park (Park hrs)
	Civic Centre Bus Station (Daytime)
	Tommyfield Market (Daytime)
	'Squire Knott', Yorkshire Street *(JDW)*
	'Up Steps Inn', High Street *(JDW)*
Royton	Shopping Precinct (Daytime)
Uppermill	Uppermill Park (Daytime)

Pendle

Barley	Picnic Area Car Park
Barnoldswick	Central Car Park, Fernlea Avenue
	Letcliffe Park, Manchester Road
	Victory Park, West View Close
Barrowford	Gisburn Road/Church Road
Brierfield	Town Hall, Colne Road (8.00-18.00)
Colne	Bus Station, Craddock Road
	Market Hall, Market Street (Market hrs)

Manchester City Council

For more information on Public Facilities and Access at many attractions, why not telephone for more details before you travel?

Please telephone for all enquiries:
0161 957 8315 MANCHESTER CITY COUNCIL

	'Wallace Hartley', Church Street *(JDW)*
Cotton Tree	Ball Grove Picnic Area
Earby	Bus Station (8.00-18.00) Colne Road, by Station Hotel (8.00-18.00) Sough Park, Colne Road
Laneshawbridge	Keighley Road, opp. Emmott Arms
Nelson	Market Hall, Leeds Road (Market hrs) Market Street
Newchurch	Village Centre
Salterforth	Kelbrook Lane/Earby Road
Wycoller	Wycoller Country Park *(Lancs CC)*

Preston

Deepdale	**CP**	Preston North End FC *(Private)* 'Nandos', Deepdale Retail Park *(Nandos)*
Preston		Avenham MSCP (6.30-23.30 Avenham Park Bus Station (M+F) (Station hrs) Guild Hall Concourse, 1st Floor (7.30-22.30) Kendal Street, nr Friargate/Corporation St. Lune Street. Near Mobility Centre Market Hall (Market hrs) Moor Park Lodge, Garstang Road (Events only) The Mall Preston *(Private)* Preston Station, Platform 3 & Waiting Room *(Virgin)* 'Centro Oriental Buffet', The Mall *(Private)*

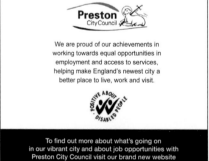
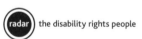

'The Greyfriar', Friargate *(JDW)*
'Wall Street', Fishergate *(Private)*
Gala Bingo Club, Market Street *(Gala)*

Ribbleton	Waverley/Ribbleton Park, Blackpool Road

Ribble Valley

Beacon Fell	Bowland Visitor Centre *(Lancs CC)*
Bolton-by-Bowland	Car Park
Chipping	Car Park
Clitheroe	Castle Field Grounds
	Church Walk
	Edisford, Riverside
	Market
	Waddington Road Cemetery
	Clitheroe Station *(Northern Rail)*
Downham	Car Park
Dunsop Bridge	Car Park
Gisburn	Auction Mart
Hurst Green	St Paul's Club
Longridge	King Street
	Berry Lane
Mellor	Mellor Lane
Ribchester	Car Park
Sabden	Car Park

Midas Mobility

Are pleased to support the
Royal Association for Disability Rights

Slaidburn	Car Park
Whalley	King Street
	Springwood Picnic Site *(Lancs CC)*

Rochdale

Greenfield	Dunsmore Reservoir *(Utd Utilities)*
Heywood	Bamford Road
	'Edwin Waugh', Market Street *(JDW)*
Heywood M62	Birch Services, J18/19 M62 *(Moto)*
Hollingworth Lake	Lakebank (Daytime)
	Pavilion Café (Café hrs)
	Visitor Centre (Centre hrs)
	'Millers', Hollingworth Lake *(Private)*
Littleborough	The Square
Middleton	Bus Station *(GMPTE)*
	'Harbord Harbord', Long Street *(JDW)*
Ogden Reservoir	Ogden Car Park *(Utd Utilities)*
Rochdale	Bus Station
	Rochdale Exchange, Market Hall subway
	South Parade
	Wheatsheaf Centre (2) *(Private)*
	'Regal Moon', The Butts *(JDW)*
Whitworth	Cowm Reservoir *(Utd Utilities)*

Rossendale

Dunnockshaw	Clowbridge Reservoir *(Utd Utilities)*
Haslingden Grane	Clough Head Inf. Centre *(Utd Utilities)*
Rawtenstall	The Market, Newchurch Road
	'Old Cobblers Inn', New Hall Hey Rd *(Private)*

St Helens

Bold Heath	'Griffin Inn', Warrington Road *(Private)*
Eccleston	'Royal Oak', East Lancashire Road *(Private)*
Garswood	Garswood Station *(Northern Rail)*
Rainford	'Bottle & Glass Inn', St Helens Road *(Private)*
St Helens	Brook Street (M+F) (Mon-Sat 9.00-18.00)

Bus Station, Bickerstaffe Street *(Merseytravel)*
St Mary's Arcade *(Private)*
'Carr Mill', East Lancashire Road *(Private)*
'Glass House', Market Street *(JDW)*
'Sefton Arms', Baldwin Street *(Private)*

Salford

Eccles	Eccles Gateway Centre (Centre hrs) Eccles Metrolink/Bus Interchange 'Albert Edward', Church Street *(Private)* 'Blue Bell', Monton Green *(Private)* 'Eccles Cross', Regent Street *(JDW)* 'White Horse', Gilda Brook Road *(Private)*
Irlam	Tesco Store, Fairhills Ind. Estate *(Tesco)* 'Railway Inn', Liverpool Road *(Private)*
Peel Green	Eccles Rugby Club *(Private)*
Salford	Salford Museum & Gallery (Museum hrs) Mothercare, West One Retail Park *(Private)* Salford Central Station *(Northern Rail)* Salford Crescent Station *(Northern Rail)* 'Quay House Beefeater' The Quays *(Private)* Fit City Clarendon, Liverpool Street *(Private)* Salford City Reds Stadium, Willows Road *(RFLC)*
Swinton	Pendleton Gateway Centre (Centre hrs) Salford Shopping City *(Private)* Victoria Park, Pavilion *(Pavilion hrs)* 'New Ellesmere', East Lancs Road *(Private)* 'Swinton Free House', Chorley Road *(Private)*
Walkden	Walkden Gateway Centre (Centre hrs) Tesco Store, Ellesmere Shopping Centre *(Tesco)*
Worsley	'Barton Arms', Stable Fold *(Private)* 'Moorings', Quayside Close, Boothstown *(Private)* Fit City Worsley Pool, Bridgewater Road *(Private)*

Sefton

Ainsdale	'The Railway', Liverpool Road *(Private)*
Blundellsands	Burbo Bank
Bootle	Bootle Bus Station *(Merseytravel)*

	New Strand Shopping Centre *(Private)*
	'Merton Inn', Merton Road *(JDW)*
	'The Wild Rose', Triad Centre *(JDW)*
	'Yates's Bar', Triad Centre *(Yates)*
Churchtown	Preston New Road
Crosby	Moor Lane
Formby	Freshfield Car Park *(National Trust)*
Maghull	Leighton Avenue
	'Coach & Horses', Liverpool Rd North *(Private)*
Southport	Eastbank Street
	Hill Street
	Market Street (09.00-17.00)
	Park Crescent, Hesketh Bank
	Promenade Central
	Ocean Plaza, Marine Drive *(Private)*
	Pleasureland (5) *(Private)*
	'Nandos', 7 Ocean Plaza *(Nandos)*
	'Sir Henry Segrave', Lord Street *(JDW)*
	'Willow Grove', Lord Street *(JDW)*
	Tony Leigh Building, Southport College *(College)*
	Esplanade Caravan Club Site *(Caravan Club)*
Waterloo	Waterloo Interchange, South Road

South Lakeland

Aldingham	Church Car Park, Foreshore
Ambleside	Mechanics Institute (Daytime)
	Rothay Park (March-November)
	Rydal Road Car Park
Arnside	Promenade Shelter
Broughton-in-Furness	The Square
Brown Howe	South of Torver, nr. Lake Coniston *(Lake District NP)*
Cark-in-Cartmell	[No specific information available]
Coniston	Park Coppice Caravan Club Site *(Caravan Club)*
Dent	Car Park *(Parish Council)*
Flookburgh	Main Street
Grange-over-Sands	Berners Close Car Park

Fernleigh Road

Meathop Fell Caravan Club Site *(Caravan Club)*

Grasmere	Moss Parrock, Village Centre
Kendal	New Road Car Park
	Peppercorn Lane
	'Miles Thompson', Allhallows Lane *(JDW)*
Kirkby Lonsdale	Jingling Lane
Milnthorpe	The Square
Monk Coniston	North end of Lake *(Lake District NP)*
Oxenholme	Oxenholm Station, Platform 1 *(Virgin)*
Sedbergh	Market Place, Joss Lane
Sedgwick	Low Park Wood Caravan Club Site *(Caravan Club)*
Staveley	Abbey Square
Ulverston	Brogden Street (Daytime)
	Canal Foot, Estuary Shore
	Croftlands/Priory Road (Daytime)
	Gill Car Park (Daytime)
	Market Hall (Daytime, not Wednesday or Sunday)
Windermere	Baddeley Clock
	Bowness Bay, Glebe Road
	Braithwaite Fold Car Park (Mid March-Oct)
	Broad Street Car Park
	Ferry Nab Car Park
	Rayrigg Road Car Park
	Braithwaite Fold Caravan Club Site *(Caravan Club)*
	White Cross Bay Leisure Park *(Private)*

South Ribble

Bamber Bridge	Withy Grove, by Supermarket (Daytime)
	'Millers', Lostock Lane *(Private)*
Lostock Hall	Hope Terrace, behind shops (Daytime)

Stockport

Bramhall	Ack Lane East
	Village Square, Ack Lane *(Private)*
	Bramhall Station *(Northern Rail)*
	'Bubble Room', Ack Lane East *(Private)*

	'Nappa Lounge Bar', Branhall Lane *(Private)*
Cheadle	Massie Street Car Park
	'Bar SH', High Street *(Private)*
	'Queens Arms', Stockport Road *(Private)*
	'The Weavers', Gatley Road *(Private)*
Cheadle Hulme	'John Millington', Station Road *(Private)*
	'Kings Hall', Station Road *(JDW)*
Compstall	Etheron Park Café, George St *(Private)*
Edgeley	Alexandra Park (Park hrs)
	Bulkeley Road
	Edgeley Library (Library hrs)
Great Moor	Great Moor Library (Library hrs)
Hazel Grove	Hazel Grove Library (Library hrs)
	Lyme Street
	Torkington Park
	'Fiveways Hotel', Macclesfield Rd *(Private)*
	'Phoenix', London Road *(Greene King)*
	'Wilfred Wood', London Road *(JDW)*
Heald Green	Heald Green Library (Library hrs)
	'Griffin', Wilmslow Road *(Holts)*
Heaton Moor	Thornfield Park (Park hrs)
	'Elizabethan', Heaton Moor Lane *(Private)*
	'Moortop', Heaton Moor Road *(Private)*
High Lane	High Lane Library (Library hrs)
Marple	Derby Street, Car Park
	Marple Library (Library hrs)
	Memorial Park
	Old Know Road
	Rose Hill
Offorton	Dialstone Centre, Lisburn Lane (Centre hrs)
Reddish	Reddish Road
	Reddish Library (Library hrs)
	'Carousel', Reddish Road *(Private)*
Romiley	Forum Car Park, Compsall Road
Stockport	Bridgefield Street
	Bus Station, Daw Bank

Vernon Park, Turncroft Lane (Park hrs)
Merseyway Shopping Centre *(Private)*
Debenhams Store, Princes Street *(Debenhams)*
Sunwin Store, Chestergate *(Private)*
Stockport Station *(Virgin)*
Stockport College, Town Centre Campus *(College)*
'Calverts Court', St Petersgate *(JDW)*
'Chestergate Tavern', Mersey Square *(Private)*
'George & Dragon', Manchester Road *(Private)*
'Pizza Hut', Wellington Road *(Private)*
'Toby Carvery', Wellington Road *(Private)*
Grand Central Swimming Pool (Pool hrs) *(Private)*

Woodley	Woodley Precinct

Tameside

Ashton-under-Lyne	Market Hall, Market Square (Hall hrs)
	Ashton Bus Station *(GMPTE)*
	Ashton-under-Lyne Station *(Northern Rail)*
	'Ash Tree', Wellington Road *(JDW)*
	'Nandos', Ashton Leisure Park *(Nandos)*
	Elysium Centre, Beaufort Road *(Tameside College)*
	Gala Bingo, Wellington Road *(Gala)*
Denton	Albert Street, by Market
	Festival Hall (Hall hrs)
Droylsden	Market Street/Greenside Lane
Hyde	Clarendon Square (Shopping hrs)
	Hyde Bus Station *(GMPTE)*
	'Cotton Bale', Market Place *(JDW)*
Mossley	Market Ground, Stamford Street
Mottram	'Mottram Wood', Stockport Road *(Private)*

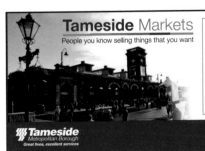

| Stalybridge | Armentieres Square, Trinity Street |
| | 'Society Rooms', Grosvenor Street *(JDW)* |

Trafford

Altrincham	Halecroft Park (Park hrs)
	John Leigh Park (Park Hrs)
	Regent Road Car Park (Mon-Sat, 9.15-17.30)
	Stamford Park (Park hrs)
	'The Unicorn', Ashley Road *(JDW)*
Bowden	'Griffin', Stamford Road *(Private)*
Dunham Massey	'Axe & Cleaver', School Lane *(Private)*
Hale	Cecil Road, Car Park (9.00-17.00)
Sale	Hereford Street (9.15-17.30)
	Woodheys Park (Park hrs)
	Worthington Park (Park hrs)
	'Cape', Waterside Plaza *(Private)*
	'Deckers', Sale Water Park (Private)
	'J P Joule', Northenden Road *(JDW)*
	'Sale Hotel', Marsland Road *(Private)*
Stretford	Longford Park (Park hrs)
	'Bishop Blaize', Chester Road *(JDW)*
	'KFC', Castlemore Retail Park *(KFC)*
	'Robin Hood', Barton Road *(Private)*
Trafford Centre **CP**	Trafford Centre (2) *(Private)*
	Barton Square *(Private)*
	Debenhams Store, Regent Cres *(Debenhams)*
	'Exchange Bar & Grill', The Orient *(Private)*
	'Ha! Ha! Bar', The Orient *(Private)*
	'Nandos', 15 The Orient *(Nandos)*
	'Rice Flamebar', The Orient *(Private)*
	'Tampopo', The Orient *(Private)*
	'TGI Fridays', The Orient *(Private)*
Trafford Park	3rd Avenue (9.00-17.00)
	'Castle in the Air', Chill Factore Centre *(JDW)*
	'Nandos', The Chill Factore *(Nandos)*
Urmston	Moorfield Walk (9.15-17.30)
	'Chadwick', Flixton Road *(Private)*
	'Tim Bobbin', Flixton Road *(JDW)*

Warrington

Birchwood		Birchwood Shopping Centre *(Private)*
		Birchwood Station *(Transpennine)*
Higher Walton	CP	Walton Hall Gardens, Park Entrance
		'Walton Arms', Old Chester Road *(Private)*
Latchford		Latchford Village
Lymm		Church Green
		Pepper Street
Lymm M6		Lymm Services J20 M6 *(Moto)*
Stockton Heath		'Nandos', 109 London Road *(Nandos)*
Stretton		'Cat & Lion', Tarporley Road *(Private)*
		'Hollow Tree', Tarporley Road *(Private)*
Warburton		'Saracens Head', Paddock Lane *(Private)*
Warrington	CP	Warrington Bus Station (8.30-23.00 Mon-Sat)
		Golden Square MSCP *(Private)*
		Golden Square Centre *(Private)*
		Lyme Street *(Private)*
		Warrington Bank Quay Station, Platform 2 *(Virgin)*
		'Friar Penketh', Barbauld Street *(JDW)*
		'Looking Glass', Buttermarket Street *(JDW)*
		'Nandos', Old Market Square *(Nandos)*
		Gala Bingo, Cockhedge Centre *(Gala)*
Winwick		'Swan', Golborne Road *(Private)*

West Lancashire

Burscough		School Lane, Car Park
Ormskirk	CP	Bus/Rail Interchange
		Church Walks
		Moor Street
		Moorgate, opp. Indoor Market
		Park Road, in Park
		Shopmobility Office, Park Road *(Private)*
Parbold		Parbold Station *(Northern Rail)*
Skelmersdale		Concourse Shopping Centre (2) *(Private)*
Tarleton		Church Road, Car Park

Wigan

Ashton-in-Makerfield	Princess Road (8.00-17.00)
	'Bay Horse', Warrington Road *(Private)*
	'Sir Thomas Gerard', Gerard Street *(JDW)*
Billinge	Winstanley College (6) *(College)*
Goose Green	'Venture', Billinge Road *(Private)*
Leigh	Bengal Street (8.00-17.00)
	Bus Station, King Street (8.00-17.00)
	'Thomas Burke', Leigh Road *(JDW)*
CP	Leigh Sports Village, Sale Road (Centre hrs)
Standish	'Charnley Arms', Almond Brook Road *(Private)*
Wigan	Bus Station, Hallgate
	Town Hall (8.45-16.30)
	The Galleries, Hindley Walk *(Private)*
	Grand Arcade Shopping Centre *(Private)*
	Wigan North Western Station, Subway *(Virgin)*
	Wigan Wallgate Station *(Northern Rail)*
	'Brocket Arms', Mesnes Road *(JDW)*
	'Moon Under Water', Market Place *(JDW)*
	'Walkabout', King Street *(Private)*
	Gala Bingo, Robin Park *(Gala)*
	Robin Park Sports Complex *(Private)*
Worthington Lakes	Visitor Centre *(Utd Utilities)*

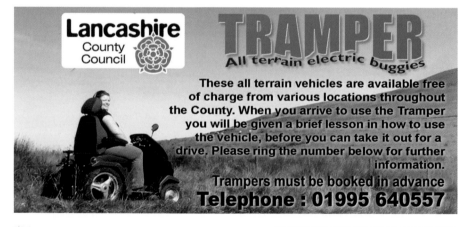

Wirral

Bebington	Bebington Civic Centre (Centre hrs)
	Bebington One Stop Shop (Office hrs)
	Higher Bebington Library (Library hrs)
Birkenhead	Cheshire Lines Building (Office hrs)
	Claughton Road Bus Station
	Conway One Stop Shop (Office hrs)
	Shopmobility Centre
	Westminster House (Office hrs)
	Woodside Bus Station
	Birkenhead Park Station *(Merseyrail)*
	'Brass Balance', Argyle Street *(JDW)*
	'John Laird', Europa Centre *(JDW)*
	Conway Park Campus *(Wirral Met College)*
	Twelve Quays Campus *(Wirral Met College)*
Bromborough	Bromborough Civic Centre (Centre hrs)
	Gala Bingo, Wirral Leisureland *(Gala)*
Eastham	Eastham Country Park
	Eastham One Stop Shop (Office hrs)
	Callett Park Campus, West Building *(Wirral Met College)*
Heswall	Heswall Library & One Stop Shop (Office hrs)
Hoylake	Hoylake Station
	Meols Parade Gardens, by bowling green
	'Hoylake Lights', Market Street *(JDW)*
Greasby	Greasby Library (Library hrs)
Irby	Irby Library (Library hrs)
Meols	Bennetts Lane, Meols Parade
Moreton	Leasowe Common
	Moreton Cross, Garden Lane
	Moreton One Stop Shop (Office hrs)
	'Grange', Hoylake Road *(Private)*
	'Mockbeggar Hall', Hoylake Road *(JDW)*
New Brighton	Harrison Drive
	New Brighton One Stop Shop (Office hrs)
New Ferry	Woodhead Street Car Park
	'John Masefield' *(JDW)*

Prenton	Prenton Library (Library hrs)
	CP Prenton Park Stadium *(Traqnmere Rovers)*
Rock Ferry	Rock Ferry One Stop Shop (Office hrs)
Thornton Hough	Thornton Common Road
Thurstaston	Wirral Country Park Visitor Centre (Centre hrs)
	Wirral Country Park Caravan Club Site *(Caravan Club)*
Upton	Upton Library (Library hrs)
Wallasey	Cherrytree Centre (Centre hrs)
	Shopmobilty Centre (Centre hrs)
	Liscard One Stop Shop (Office hrs)
	Seacombe Library (Library hrs)
	Wallasey Central Library (Library hrs)
	Wallasey Town Hall (Office hrs)
	'Clairville', Wallasey Road *(JDW)*
West Kirby	Dee Lane, West Kirby Lakes
	Grange Road, by Station
	West Kirby Concourse (Centre hrs)
	'Dee Hotel', Grange Road *(JDW)*
Woodchurch	Landican Cemetery (Cemetery hrs)
	Woodchurch Library (Library hrs)

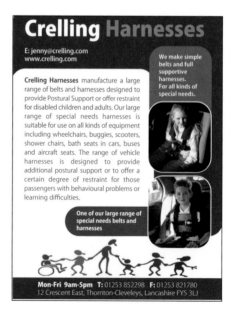

Wyre

Fleetwood	Beach Road, by Cemetery
	Bold Street, Euston Park
	Marine Hall Car Park
	Preston Street
	'Thomas Drummond', London St *(JDW)*
Garstang	High Street, Community Centre Car Park
	Park Hill Road Car Park
Great Eccleston	The Weind, off High Street
Knott End	Barton Square
	The Ferry
Pilling	School Lane
Poulton	Teanlowe Centre, Queensway
CP	United Reformed Church, Titebarn Street *(Church)*
	Poulton-le-Fylde Station *(Northern Rail)*
Scorton	Gubberford Lane
Thornton Cleveleys	Rough Lea Road, Car Park
	North Drive
	Shopping Precinct, Victoria Rd East
	Wyre Estuary Country Park, Visitor Centre

Barnsley

Barnsley	Cheapside, nr Market Hall
CP	Barnsley Town Hall (Office hrs)
	Metropolitan Shopping Centre *(Private)*
	Barnsley Station *(SYPTE)*
	'Escapade', Wellington Street (2) *(Private)*
	'Heart of Barnsley', Peel Street *(Marstons)*
	'Joseph Brammahs', Market Hill *(JDW)*
	'Silkstone Inn', Market Street *(JDW)*
	'Walkabout', Church Street *(Private)*
	'White Bear', Church Street *(Private)*
	Parkway Cinema, Eldon Street *(Private)*
Cudworth	'Fayre & Square', Darfield Road *(Private)*
Monk Bretton	'Norman Inn', Burton Road *(Private)*
Wombwell	'The Horseshoe', High Street *(JDW)*

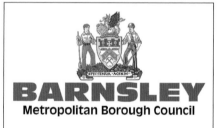

Bradford

Bingley		Market, Chapel Lane 'Midland Hotel', Main Street *(Private)* 'Myrtle Grove', Main Street *(JDW)*
Bradford	**CP**	Bradford Central Library (Library hrs) City Hall, Bradford Centre (M+F) Lister Park (Park hrs) Centenary Square (Private) Kirkgate Shopping Centre *(Private)* Oastler Shopping Centre *(Private)* Ladbrokes, Lillycroft Road *(Private)* Bradford Interchange Bus Station *(WYMetro)* Bradford Forster Sq. Station *(Northern Rail)* 'Bar:Me', Great Horton Rd *(Private)* 'City Vaults', Hustlergate *(Private)* 'Goose on Bridge Street', Bridge Street *(M&B)* 'Manor House', Leeds Road *(Private)* 'Markaz Restaurant', Cemtenary Sq *(Private)* 'Nandos', The Leisure Exchange *(Nandos)* 'Sir Titus Salt', Morley Street *(JDW)* 'Turls Green', Centenary Square *(JDW)* 'Unicorn', Ivegate *(Private)* 'Varsity', Great Horton St *(Barracuda)* Gala Bingo, Tong Street *(Gala)*
	CP	Carlisle Business Centre *(Private)* Bradford College, Gt. Horton Street *(College)*
	CP	Mind the Gap Studios, Patent Street *(Private)*
	CP	University of Bradford, Richmond Building *(University)*
Burley-in-Wharfedale		Station Road
East Bowling	**CP**	Bowling Pool, Flockton Road
Eccleshill	**CP**	Eccleshill Leisure Centre, Harrogate Road
Esholt		Car Park, Station Road
Guiseley		Guiseley Station *(Northern Rail)*
Harden		St Ives Estate Car Park
Haworth		Bronte Parsonage Car Park (M+F) Central Park, Rawdon Road Penistone Hill Country Park (M+F) (Summer)
Idle		'Hitching Post', Leeds Road *(Marstons)*

Ilkley		Central Car Park, Brooke Street
		Riverside, Bridge House Lane (M+F)
		White Wells
	CP	Ilkley Pool & Lido
Keighley		Cavendish Street
		Keighley Market
	CP	Keighley Leisure Centre
		Bus Station, Towngate *(WYMetro)*
		'Livery Rooms', North Street *(JDW)*
		Gala Bingo, Alice Street *(Gala)*
		Keighley Bowl, Alston Retail Park *(Private)*
Menston		'Hare & Hounds', Bradford Road *(Private)*
Odsall		Grattan Stadium *(Bradford Bulls)*
Saltaire		Caroline Street (M+F)
Shipley		Market Square
		'Lloyds Bar', Market Square *(JDW)*
Silsden		Car Park, Bridge Street
Thornbury		'The Farmers', Bradford Road *(Private)*
Thornton	**CP**	Thornton Recreation Centre
Wibsey		'Ancient Foresters', High Street *(Private)*
Wilsden		'Prune Park Bar' *(Private)*

Calderdale

Brighouse	Brighouse Library (Library hrs)
	Rastrick Library (Library hrs)
	Thornton Square
	'Richard Ostler', Bethal Street *(JDW)*
	Holiday Inn Health Club, Clifton Village *(Private)*
Elland	Town Hall Square
Halifax	Albion Street (Mon-Sat, daytime)
	Borough Market (Market hrs)
	George Square
	Manor Heath Park
	North Bridge Leisure Centre (Centre hrs)
	Ogden Water Country Park
	People's Park
	Piece Hall (2) (Daytime)

Savile Park, Skircoat
Halifax Bus Station *(WYMetro)*
Halifax Station, Platform 2 *(Northern Rail)*
'Barun Top Inn', Rawson Street *(JDW)*
'Caffe Nero', Southgate *(Caffe Nero)*
'Flutter Bites', Manor Heath Park *(Private)*
'Goose at the Arcade', Commercial Street *(M&B)*
'Millers', Salterhebble Hill *(Private)*
'Salvation', Bull Green *(Barracuda)*
Reception, Calderdale College, Francis Street *(College)*
The Shay Stadium (2) *(Halifax Town FC)*

Hebden Bridge	Calder Holmes Park (Summer, Park hrs)
	New Road
	Valley Road
	Hebden Bridge Station *(Northern Rail)*
Heptonstall	Towngate Car Park
Luddenden	Luddenden Lane
Mytholmroyd	Bridge End
Ripponden	Brig Royd

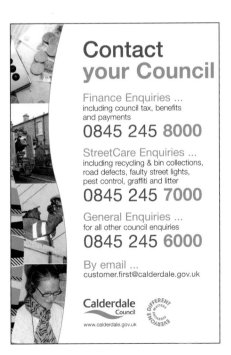

Contact your Council

Finance Enquiries ...
including council tax, benefits
and payments

0845 245 8000

StreetCare Enquiries ...
including recycling & bin collections,
road defects, faulty street lights,
pest control, graffiti and litter

0845 245 7000

General Enquiries ...
for all other council enquiries

0845 245 6000

By email ...
customer.first@calderdale.gov.uk

Calderdale
Council

www.calderdale.gov.uk

Trevor Smith Property

Are pleased to support the Royal Association for Disability Rights

Sowerby Bridge	Wharf Street Car Park
Shibden	Mereside Centre, Shibden Park (Centre hrs) Shibden Hall (10.00-16.30) Shibden Park Playground (Park hrs)
Todmorden	Brook Street Centre Vale Park, South Lodge (Daytime)

Craven

Bolton Abbey	Strid Wood Caravan Club Site *(Caravan Club)*
Buckden	Car Park *(Yorks. Dales NP)*
Clapham	Car Park *(Yorks. Dales NP)*
Cowling	Keighley Road
Gargrave	High Street/South Street (Dawn-Dusk)
Glusburn	Main Street
Grassington	Car Park *(Yorks. Dales NP)*
High Bentham	Main Car Park
Horton-in-Ribblesdale	Car Park *(Yorks. Dales NP)*
Ingleton	Community Centre Car Park *(Parish Council)*
Kettlewell	Car Park *(Yorks. Dales NP)*
Malham	Car Park *(Yorks. Dales NP)*
Settle	Ashfield Car Park Whitefriars Car Park, Church Street
Skipton	Bus Station Coach Street Car Park Town Hall (Office hrs) Skipton Station (2) *(Northern Rail)*

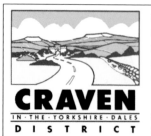

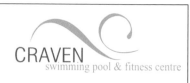

Swimming Pools
Large Fitness Centre
Coffee Lounge
Studio Excercise Classes
Tennis /Golf

Full Disabled Access
Large Free Customer Car Park

Aireville Park, Skipton,
North Yorkshire,
BD23 1UD
Tel: 01756 792 805

	'Devonshire', Newmarket Street *(JDW)*
CP	South Skipton Day Service (Centtre hrs)
Stainforth	Car Park *(Yorks. Dales NP)*
Threshfield	Wharfedale Caravan Club Site *(Caravan Club)*

Doncaster

Adwick	Adwick Station *(Northern Rail)*
Bawtry	Gainsborough Road
Bentley	Bentley Park Gates, Cooke Street
Conisbrough	Church Street
Doncaster	Council House, College Rd (Office hrs) Market Place, High Fishergate (7.00-17.00) Southern Bus Station (7.30-17.30) Frenchgate Centre (11) *(Private)* Doncaster Station, Platform 8&3A *(East Coast)* 'Che Bar', Silver Street *(Private)* 'Gatehouse', Priory Walk *(JDW)* 'Old Angel', Cleveland Street *(JDW)* 'Red Lion', Market Place *(JDW)* 'Walkabout', Priory Walk *(Private)*
Hatfield M18	Doncaster North Services, J5 M18 *(Moto)*
High Melton	Doncaster College, University Centre *(College)*
Mexborough	Market Street, opp. Fish Market 'Old Market Hall', Market Street *(JDW)*
Moorends	Wembley Road
Thorne	The Green, Finkle Street
Tickhill	The Library (Library hrs)

East Riding Of Yorkshire

Beverley	Dyer Lane (Daytime) Lord Roberts Road (Daytime) Sow Hill Bus Station (Daytime) Station Square
Bridlington	Beaconsfield Promenade (Daytime) Belvedere Parade, Boat Compound (Summer) Coach Park, Hilderthorpe Road (Daytime)

Limekiln Lane (Daytime)
Princess Mary Promenade (Daytime)
Queen Street
Royal Princess Parade (Daytime)
CP South Cliff Gardens
South Marine Drive (Summer, daytime)
The Promenades *(Private)*
Bridlington Station *(Northern Rail)*
'Prior John', Promenade *(JDW)*
Gala Bingo, Promenade *(Gala)*

Brough	'Ferry Inn', Station Road *(Marstons)*
Cottingham	Market Green (Daytime)
Driffield	Cross Hill *(Town Council)*
	North Street *(Town Council)*
	CP Driffield Leisure Centre (Centre hrs)
Flamborough	Lighthouse (Daytime)
Goole	Escourt Street (Daytime)
	'City & County', Market Square *(JDW)*
Hedon	Watmoughs Arcade (Daytime)

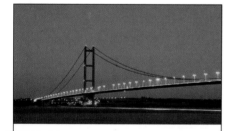

The Humber Bridge

A masterpiece of civil engineering, and one of the world's longest single span suspension bridges (1,410 metres), the Humber Bridge is an attraction in its own right and well worth a visit before continuing your journey to the other attractions in the region.

For information on tolls, discounts, and toll exemption
Telephone: 01482 647 161

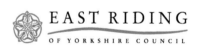

EAST RIDING
OF YORKSHIRE COUNCIL

For more information on public facilities and access at many attractions, why not telephone for more details before you travel?

Please telephone for all enquires: 01482 393939

Hessle	Cliff Road, Hessle Mill (Daytime)
	The Square (Daytime)
	Humber Bridge Car Park *(Bridge Board)*
Hornsea	Boat Compound (Summer)
	Cinema Street (Daytime)
	Marine Drive (Daytime)
Howden	St Helens Square (Daytime)
Kilnsea	Seaside Road Car Park (Daytime)
Mappleton	Cliff Road Car Park (Daytime)
Market Weighton	Londesborough Road (Daytime)
North Ferriby	'Duke of Cumberland', High St. *(Marstons)*
Pocklington	Railway Street (Daytime)
	CP Francis Scaife Sports Centre (Centre hrs)
Sewerby	Sewerby Park (Summer)
	Sewerby Cricket Club, by Pavilion (Daytime)
Stamford Bridge	The Square
Withernsea	Central Promenade (Daytime)
	Piggy Lane (Daytime)

Hambleton

Bedale	Bridge Street Car Park
Chopgate	Car Park *(North York Moors NP)*
Easingwold	Market Place
Great Ayton	Park Rise, off High Street
Kildale	Kildale Station
	Car Park *(North York Moors NP)*
Northallerton	Applegarth Car Park (8.00-19.00)
	CP Chopsticks Workshop & Resource Centre *(Private)*
	CP Hambleton Forum, Bullamore Rd (Centre hrs)
	CP Northdale Horticulture, Yafforth Rd *(Private)*
Osmotherly	South End/School Lane
Stokesley	High Street
Sutton Bank	Visitor Centre *(North York Moors NP)*
Swainby	[No specific information available]
Thirsk	Market Place
	Millgate Car Park

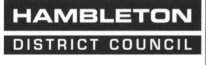

SUPPORTS THE RADAR NATIONAL KEY SCHEME

Keys are available to purchase at:

Council Offices:
Civic Centre, Stonecross, Northallerton.
Area Office, College Square, Stokesley.
Area Office, Manor Road, Easingwold.

Tourist Information Centres:
Northallerton - Applegarth Car Park
Thirsk - 49 Market Place
Great Ayton - High Green Car Park
Easingwold - Chapel Lane
Bedale - Bedale Hall, North End

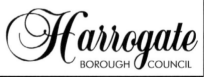

Working for you

Supports the
RADAR National Key Scheme
Keys are available to purchase at:
Council Offices:
Crescent Gardens, Harrogate.
Knapping Mount, Harrogate.
Springfield Avenue, Harrogate.
Shopmobility Unit. (Car Park level 10), Victoria.
Multi-Storey Car Park, Harrogate.
Housing Needs Office, Victoria Avenue, Harrogate.
High Street, Knaresborough House
Town Hall, Market Place, Ripon.

Tourist Information Centres:
Pateley Bridge, High Street.
Harrogate - Royal Baths, Crescent Gardens.
Knaresborough - off Market Place.
Ripon - Opposite Minster.
Boroughbridge - High Street

CP Thirsk Leisure Centre (Centre hrs)
Thirsk Station *(Transpennine)*
'Three Tuns', Market Place *(JDW)*

Harrogate

Beckwithshaw	'Smiths Arms', Church Row *(Private)*
Boroughbridge	Back Lane Car Park
Harrogate	Crescent Gardens, Crescent Road
	Devonshire Place, Skipton Road

CP Harrogate Library (Library hrs)
Hydro Swimming Pool (Pool hrs)
Jubilee MSCP
Library Gardens, Victoria Avenue
Oatlands Recreation Ground, Hookstone Rd
Starbeck High Street
Stray Ponds, York Place
Tower Street MSCP
Valley Gardens
Victoria MSCP
Victoria Shopping Centre *(Private)*

Harrogate Station *(Northern Rail)*
Asda Store, Bower Road *(Asda)*
'Winter Gardens', Royal Baths *(JDW)*

Knaresborough	Bond End, High Street
	Bus Station
	Castle Yard
	Conyngham Hall Car Park
	York Place Car Park
	Knaresborough Caravan Club Site *(Caravan Club)*
	CP Gracious Street Methodist Church Centre *(Private)*
	CP Henshaws Arts & Crafts Centre *(Private)*
	CP Knaresborough Swimming Pool (Pool hrs)
Masham	Dixon Keld, nr. Police Station
Pateley Bridge	Recreation Ground
	Southlands Car Park
Ripley	Visitors Car Park
Ripon	Bus Station
	Minster Road
	Spa Gardens
	Wakemans House, High Skellgate
Sickinghall	'Scotts Arms', Main Street *(Private)*

Kingston-Upon-Hull

Hull	Albert Avenue Pools (Centre hrs)
	Costello Athletics Stadium (Stadium hrs)
	Guildhall Square
	Holderness Road, by East Park
	Hull Arena (Arena hrs)
	Hull Central Library (Library hrs)
	West Park (Park hrs)
	Woodford Leisure (Centre hrs)
	CP Goodwin Centre, Guildhall Road (Centre hrs)
	North Point Shopping Centre *(Private)*
	Princes Quay Shopping Centre *(Private)*
	Prospect Shopping Centre *(Private)*
	CP St Stephens Shopping Centre *(Private)*
	Trinity Market. North Church Side *(Private)*
	Debenhams Store, Prospect St. *(Debenhams)*
	'Admiral of the Humber', Anlaby Rd *(JDW)*

'Apollo', Holderness High Road *(Marstons)*
'Bridges', Suitton Road *(Private)*
'Biarritz', George Street *(Marstons)*
'Goodfellowship', Cottingham Rd *(Marstons)*
'Highway', Willerby Road *(Marstons)*
'Hog's Head', Whitefriargate *(Private)*
'Hull Cheese', Paragon Street *(Private)*
'Linnet & Lark', Princess Ave *(Marstons)*
'Lyrics', Whitefriargate *(Private)*
'Mainbrace', Beverley Road *(Private)*
'Nandos', St Stephens Centre *(Nando)*
'Oystercatcher', Kingswood Leisure Park *(Private)*
'Parkers', Anlaby Road *(Private)*
'Priory Inn', Priory Road *(Marstons)*
'Revolution', Lowgate *(Private)*
'Sutton Fields', Oslo Road *(M&B)*
'3 John Scotts', Alfred Gelder Street *(JDW)*
'White Horse', Carr Lane *(Private)*
'William Wilberforce', Trinity House Lane *(JDW)*
'Zachariah Pearson', Beverley Road *(JDW)*
Gala Bingo, Oslo Road *(Gala)*
Mecca Bingo, Anlaby Road *(Mecca)*
Odeon Cinema, Kingston Retail Park *(Odeon)*

Kirklees

Batley	Batley Town Hall (Office hrs)
	Market Square
	Wilton Park (Park hrs)
	'Union Rooms', Hick Lane *(JDW)*
Birstall	Oakwell Hall Information Centre
	Town Centre
	'Nandos', Junct 27 M62, Gelderd Road *(Nandos)*
Cleckheaton	Cleckheaton Town Hall (Office hrs)
	Market Arcade
	'Obediah Brooke', Bradford Road *(JDW)*
Dalton	Rawthorne & Dalton Library, Ridgeway (Library hrs)
Dewsbury	Crow Nest Park (Park hrs)
	Dewsbury Library (Library hrs)
	Dewsbury Museum (Museum hrs)
	Dewsbury Town Hall (Office hrs)

Longcauseway, Market Place
Social Services Information Point
Dewsbury Bus Station *(WYMetro)*
'The Principle', Northgate *(Barracuda)*
'West Riding', by Station *(Private)*
'The Time Piece', Northgate *(JDW)*

Fartown   Birkby & Fartown Library (Library hrs)

Heckmondwike   Heckmondwike Market
Oldfield Lane

Holme   Village Centre

Holmfirth   Bus Station, Towngate

Honley   Moorbottom

Huddersfield   Albion Street, Civic Centre Car Park
Civic Centre 1 (Office hrs)
Greenhead Park (Park hrs)
Huddersfield Library & Art Gallery (Library hrs)
Huddersfield Covered Market
Library (Library hrs)
Queensgate Market
Town Hall (Office hrs)
The Media Centre *(Private)*
Bus Station, Albion Street *(WYMetro)*
Huddersfield Station *(Transpennine)*
Beatties Store, Kingsgate Centre *(Private)*
'Caffe Nero', King Street *(Caffe Nero)*
'Cherry Tree', John William Street *(JDW)*
'Old Court House', Queens Street *(Private)*
'Lord Wilson', King Street *(JDW)*
'Nandos', John William Street *(Nandos)*
'Varsity', Zetland Street *(Barracuda)*
'Warehouse', Zetland Street *(Private)*
'Yates's Bar', King Street *(Yates)*

Marsden   Peel Street

Marsh   Westbourne Road

Milnsbridge   Morley Lane

Mirfield   Knowle Park
Station Road
'Ship Inn', Steanant Lane *(Private)*

New Mill	Holmfirth Road
Outlane	'Waggon & Horses', New Hay Lane *(Private)*
Ravensknowle	Tolson Museum (Museum hrs)
Slaithwaite	Carr Lane

Leeds

Armley	Theaker Lane
	CP Armley Leisure Centre (Centre hrs)
Boston Spa	Village Hall, High St. *(Parish Council)*
Bramhope	Golden Acre Park (Park hrs)
	Old Lane Car Park
Beeston	Cottingley Hall Crematorium (Crematorium hrs)
Bramley	Town Street
Chapel Allerton	Scott Hall Sports Centre (Centre hrs)
	'Three Hulats', Harrogate Road *(JDW)*
Chapeltown	**CP** Reginald Centre (Centre hrs)
Crossgates	Crossgates Library (Library hrs)
	Cross Gates Shopping Centre *(Private)*
Garforth	Barleyhill Road
Gledhow	Fearnville Leisure Centre (Centre hrs)
Gildersome	Gildersome Library (Library hrs)
Headingley	Ash Road/North Lane
	Carnegie Stadium, S. Stand *(Leeds Rugby)*
	Headingley Stadium *(Yorkshire CCC)*
Holt Park	Holt Park Community Library (Library hrs)
Horsforth	Horsforth Library (Library hrs)
	Horsforth Station *(Northern Rail)*
Leeds	County Arcade, Vicar Lane
	Kirkgate Market, Vicar Lane
	St John's Centre, Albion Street/Merrion Street
	The Corn Exchange, Call Lane *(Private)*
	Headrow Shopping Centre *(Private)*
	The Light, The Headrow (2) *(Private)*
	CP Trinity Leeds *(Private)* [Planned}
	Debenhams Store, Briggate *(Debenhams)*

Debenhams Store, White Rose *(Debenhams)*
Leeds City Bus Station *(WYMetro)*
Leeds Station (3) *(Network Rail)*
West Yorkshire Playhouse *(Private)*
'Beckets Bank', Park Row *(JDW)*
'Bourbon', Cookridge Street *(Private)*
'Browns', The Headrow *(M&B)*
'The Courtyard', Cookridge Street *(Private)*
'Cuthbert Brodrick', Portland Crescent *(JDW)*
'Edwards', Merrion Street *(M&B)*
'Ha! Ha! Bar', Millennium Square *(Private)*
'Hedley Verity', Woodhouse Lane *(JDW)*
'Hog's Head', Great George Street *(Private)*
'J D Wetherpoon', Leeds Station *(JDW)*
'Japanic', Clay Pit Lane *(Private)*
'Jongleurs', The Cube *(Private)*
'Majestyk', City Square *(Private)*
'McDonalds', Briggate *(McDonalds)*
'McDonalds', St Johns Shopping Centre *(McDonalds)*
'Nandos', 152 Briggate *(Nandos)*
'Nandos', Cardigan Fields *(Nandos)*

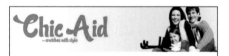

'Nandos', The Light *(Nandos)*
'Nation of Shopkeepers', Cookridge St *(Private)*
'Packhorse', Briggate *(Private)*
'Prohibition', Greek Street *(Private)*
'Qube', Portland Crescent *(Private)*
'Queens Court', Lower Briggate *(Private)*
'Quid Pro Quo', Greek Street *(Private)*
'Revolution', Cookridge Street *(Private)*
'Slug & Lettuce', Park Road *(Private)*
'Squares', Boar Lane *(Private)*
'Stick or Twist', The Podium *(JDW)*
'Tampopo', South Parade *(Private)*
'Tiger Tiger', Albion Street *(Private)*
'Varsity', Woodhouse Lane *(Barracuda)*
'Walkabout', Cookridge Street *(Private)*
'Waterhole', Great George Street *(Private)*
'The Wellington', Wellington Street *(Private)*
'Wetherspoons', City Station *(JDW)*
'Yates's Bar', Boar Lane *(Yates)*
'Yates's Bar', Woodhouse Lane *(Yates)*
Elland Road Stadium *(Leeds Utd)*
West Yorkshire Playhouse, Quarry Hill *(Private)*

Moor Allerton		'Penny Fun', Shopping Centre *(Private)*
Morley		Morley Town Hall (Office hrs)
		Wesley Street/Queen Street
	CP	Morley Leisure Centre (Centre hrs)
Osmondthorpe		Osmondthorpe Library/One Stop Centre (Centre hrs)
Otley	CP	Chevin Forest Park, by Study Centre
		Nelson Street, Visitors Centre & Library
		'Bowling Green', Bondgate *(JDW)*
Pudsey		Market Place
Rothwell		Marsh Street, Car Park
Roundhay		Tropical World (Park hrs)
Wetherby		The Shambles, Cross Street
		Wetherby Services, A1(M) Junct 46 *(Moto)*

Richmondshire

Askrigg	Village Hall (Hall hrs)
Aysgarth Falls	Car Park *(Yorks. Dales NP)*
Bainbridge	[No specific information available]
Catterick Village	Bank Yard
Colburn	Broadway
	CP Catterick Road Leisure Centre *(Private)*
Grinton	[No specific information available]
Gunnerside	[No specific information available]
Hawes	Market Place
	Car Park *(Yorks. Dales NP)*
	Brown Moor Caravan Club Site *(Caravan Club)*
Hipswell	Hildyard Row/White Shops
Keld	[No specific information available]
Langthwaite	[No specific information available]
Leyburn	Kelberdale
	Railway Street
	Lower Wesleydale Caravan Club Site *(Caravan Club)*
Middleham	[No specific information available]
Muker	[No specific information available]
Reeth	[No specific information available]
Richmond	The Falls
	Nuns Close Car Park

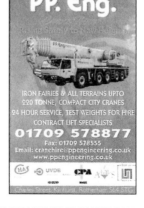

Reeth Road Cemetery
Ronaldshay Park
Round House
Victoria Road
'Ralph Fitz Randell', Queens Road *(JDW)*
Hargill House Caravan Club Site *(Caravan Club)*

Rotherham

Aston-cumAughton	Leisure Centre (Centre hrs)
East Dene	Mowbray Gardens Library (Library hrs)
Greasbrough	Greasbrough Library (Library hrs)
Maltby	Joint Customer Care Centre (Centre hrs)
	Leisure Centre (Centre hrs)
Rotherham	All Saints Square (Daytime)
	Centenary Market Hall Entrance (Market hrs)
	Clifton Park Museum, Clifton Lane (Museum hrs)
CP	Clifton Park Wet Play Area (Park hrs)
	St Ann's Leisure Centre (Centre hrs)
CP	Town Hall (Daytime)
	Rotherham Central Station *(Northern Rail)*
	'The Blue Coat', The Crofts *(JDW)*
	'Corn Law Rhymer', High Street *(JDW)*
	'The Rhinoceros', Bridgegate *(JDW)*
Thrybergh	Country Park, Anglers' Lodge
Wath-upon-Dearn	'Church House', Montgomery Square *(JDW)*

Ryedale

Danby	The Moors Centre *(North York Moors NP)*
Grosmont	Grosmont Station *(NYMR)*
Helmsley	Borogate
	Cleveland Way Car Park
Hutton-le-Hole	Car Park *(North York Moors NP)*
Kirkbymoorside	Town Farm Car Park
Malton	Market Place
	Wentworth Street
Norton	Church Street
Pickering	Eastgate

	The Ropery Car Park Pickering Station *(NYMR)*
Rosedale	Rosedale Abbey
Staxton	Saxton Brow Picnic Area
Thornton-le-Dale	Lakeside Car Park

Scarborough

Filey	The Beach (Easter-October) Ravine, Cobble Landing Royal Parade Station Avenue Car Park
Glaisdale	Station Car Park
Goathland	Car Park *(North York Moors NP)* Goathland Station *(NYMR)*
Grosmont	Front Street
Ravenscar	Raven Hall Road *(North York Moors NP)*
Robin Hood's Bay	Bank Bottom Station Car Park (Summer)
Scaling Dam	Car Park *(North York Moors NP)*
Scarborough	Burniston Road Car Park North Bay Peasholme Park Royal Albert Drive, North Bay South Cliff Gardens, nr. Spa (Easter-Oct) Sports Centre (Centre hrs) St Helens Square St Nicholas, Foreshore (Easter-Oct) West Pier Brunswick Shopping Centre *(Private)* Debenhams Store, Brunswick Pavilion *(Debenhams)* Scarborough Station, Platform 3 *(Transpennine)* 'Lord Rosebery', Westborough *(JDW)* 'The West Riding', Castle Road *(M&B)*
Staithes	Staithes Bank Bottom Staithes Top Car Park
West Ayton	West Ayton Caravan Club Site *(Caravan Club)*
Whitby	Abbey Headland, Car Park

Kyber Pass, The Battery
Marina, Car Park
New Quay, New Quay Road
North Promanade, The Beach
West Cliff Beach (Easter-Oct)
Whitby Leisure Centre

Selby

Barlow Common	Nature Reserve Visitor Centre (Centre hrs)
Selby	Abbey Leisure Centre (Centre hrs)
	Back Micklegate Car Park
	Park Street, by Selby Park
	Morrisons Store, Market Cross *(Morrison)*
	Tesco Store, Portholme Road *(Tesco)*
Sherburn-in-Elmet	Low Street
Tadcaster	Britannia Car Park

Sheffield

Beighton	'Belfry', Eckington Road *(Private)*
Broomhill	'Francis Newton', Clarkehouse Road *(JDW)*
Chapeltown	Park Gates, Cowley Lane (Daytime)
Crystal Peaks	Crystal Peaks Shopping Centre *(Private)*
Foxhouse	Public House Car Park, Hathersage Road
Gower Street	Ellesmere Road Shops
Hillsborough	'Rawson Spring', Langsett Road *(JDW)*

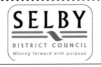

Meadowhall	Debenhams Store, Park Lane *(Debenhams)*
	Meadowhall Station *(SYPTE)*
	'Nandos', The Oasis *(Nandos)*
Norton	Main Road/Meadowhead
Rivelin	Manchester Road/Rivelin Valley Road
Sheffield City Centre	Angel Street
	Moorfoot (Mon-Sat, 7.00-18.15)
	CP Royal Hallamshire Hospital *(NHS Trust)*
	Castle Market (Market hrs) *(Private)*
	Orchard Square *(Private)*
	Debenhams Store, The Moor *(Debenhams)*
	Sheffield Station, Concourse *(E Midlands Trains)*
	Sheffield Station, Platform 5 *(E Midlands Trains)*
	'Bankers Draft', Market Place *(JDW)*
	'Benjamin Huntsman', Cambridge Street *(JDW)*
	'Ha! Ha! Bar', St Pauls Parade *(Private)*
	'Nandos', West Street *(Nandos)*
	'Sheaf Island', Ecclesall Road *(JDW)*
	'Sheffield Waterworks Co', Division St *(JDW)*
	'Swim Inn', Glossop Road *(JDW)*
	'Varsity', Eccleshall Road *(Barracuda)*
	'Varsity', West Street *(Barracuda)*
	'Walkabout', Carver Street *(Private)*
	Bramall Lane Stadium *(Sheffield Utd)*
	CP Ponds Forge, Sheaf Street *(Private)*
	CP Sheffield Town Hall (Office hrs)
Stocksbridge	Market Street

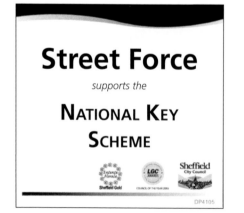

Street Force

supports the

NATIONAL KEY

SCHEME

 the disability rights people

Get Mobile

Radar's independent guide to help you purchase a mobility scooter or powered wheelchair.

Available from Radar's online shop
www.radar-shop.org.uk

Tinsley	**CP**	Tinsley Green Childrens Centre (Centre hrs)
Valley Entertainment Centre		'Nandos', Broughton Lane *(Nandos)*
Woodseats	**CP**	Abbey Lane 'Woodseats Palace', Chesterfield Rd *(JDW)*

Wakefield

Ackworth		'Beverley Arms', Doncaster Rd *(Marstons)*
Castleford		Carlton Lane Shopping Centre *(Private)* Castleford Bus Station *(WYMetro)* 'Carltons', Carlton Street *(Private)* 'Glass Blower', Bank Street *(JDW)* 'Nandos', Xscape *(Nandos)* 'Shout', Station Road *(Private)* 'Winter Seam', Xscape *(JDW)* Bowlplex, Xscape *(Private)*
Darrington		'The Darrington', Gt. North Road *(Private)*
Glasshoughton	**CP**	Junction 32 Outlet Village *(Private)*
Hemsworth		Vale Head Sports Pavilion (Centre hrs)
Horbury		Horbury Library, Westfield Rd (Library hrs) 'Old Mill', Wakefield Road *(Private)*
Knottingley M62		Ferrybridge Services, J30 M62/A1 *(Moto)*
Ossett		Ossett Town Hall (Office hrs)
Pontefract		Pontefract Town Hall (Office hrs) Pontefract Bus Station *(WYMetro)* 'Broken Bridge', Horsefair *(JDW)* 'Red Lion', Market Place *(Private)*
Wakefield		The Springs Wakefield Reference Library (Library hrs) Wakefield Town Hall (Office hrs)
	CP	The Ridings Shopping Centre (2) *(Private)* 'Caffe Nero', Kirkgate *(Private)* 'The Gate', Northgate *(Marstons)* 'Lupset Hotel', Horbury Road *(Private)* 'Nandos', Westgate Retail Park *(Nandos)* 'Quest', Westgate *(Private)* 'Six Chimneys', Kirkgate *(JDW)* 'Slug & Fiddle', Almsgate *(Private)*

| West Bretton M1 | Woolley Edge Services, J38/39 M1 *(Moto)* |

York

Acomb	Front Street (8.00-20.00)
	CP Acomb Library (Library hrs)
	CP Oaklands Leisure Centre [Planned]
	'Marcia Grey', Front Street *(Private)*
Clifton	Homestead Park (Daytime) *(Rowntree Trust)*
Dringhouses	Askham Bar Park & Ride
Fulford	York Designer Outlet *(Private)*
Grimston	Grimston Bar Park & Ride
Haxby	Town Centre (8.00-20.00)
Rawcliffe	Rawcliffe Bar Park & Ride
York	Coppergate (8.00-20.00)
	Kent Street, Car Park (8.00-20.00)
	Museum Gardens (April-Sept)
	Nunnery Lane, Car Park (8.00-20.00)
	Parliament Street (8.00-20.00)
	Rowntree Park, Terry Avenue (Park hrs)
	St George's Field (April-Sept)
	St Leonards Place, Exhibition Square (8.00-20.00)
	St Sampsons Square (8.00-20.00)
	CP Silver Street
	Tanner Row (8.00-20.00)
	Union Terrace, Car Park (8.00-20.00)
	York Central Library (Library hrs)
	CP Long Close Lane, Walmgate
	York Station, Platforms 2 & 8 *(East Coast)*
	'Ha! Ha! Bar', New Street *(Private)*
	'Loch Fyne Restaurant', Walmgate *(Private)*
	'Nandos', High Ousegate *(Nandos)*
	'Postern Gate', Piccadilly *(JDW)*
	'Punch Bowl', Blossom Street *(JDW)*
	'Royal York Hotel', Station Road *(Private)*
	'Slug & Lettuce', Low Ousegate *(Private)*
	'Varsity', 6-12 Lendal *(Barracuda)*
	'Windmill', Blossom Street *(Private)*
	'Yates's Bar', Low Ousegate *(Yates)*
	City Screen, Coney Street *(Private)*

Mecca Bingo, Fishergate *(Private)*
York City Knights Rugby Stadium *(Private)*
York Race Course *(Private)*
Beechwood Grange Caravan Club Site *(Caravan Club)*
Rowntree Park Caravan Club Site *(Caravan Club)*

NORTH EAST ENGLAND

Darlington

Darlington	Horsemarket, by Shopmobility
	Cornmill Shopping Centre *(Private)*
	Darlington Station, Platform 4 *(East Coast)*
	'The Brinkburn', Lady Katherine Grove *(Private)*
	'The Mowden', Staindrop Road *(M&B)*
	'Tanners Hall', Skinnergate *(JDW)*
	'William Stead', Crown Street *(JDW)*
	'Yates's Bar', Skinnergate *(Yates)*
	Gala Bingo, Skinnergate *(Gala)*
CP	Dolphin Centre. Horsemarket (Centre hrs)

Durham

Allensford	Allensford Caravan/Picnic Park, off A68
Barnard Castle	Galgate Car Park
	Teesdale Barnard Castle Caravan Club Site *(Caravan Club)*
Bishop Auckland	Bus Station
	'Stanley Jefferson', Market Place *(JDW)*
Chester-le-Street	Foundry Lane (Mon-Sat, 9.00-17.00)
	Riverside (Daytime)
	Chester-le-Street Station *(Northern Rail)*
	'Wicket Gate', Front Street *(JDW)*
Consett	Consett Bus Station, Medomsley Road
Crimdon	Crimdon Park
Durham	Milburngate Shopping Centre (Shopping hrs)
	Walkergate Car Park (8.00-18.00)
	Durham Station *(East Coast)*
	'Bishops Mill', Walkergate *(JDW)*
	'Hog's Head', Saddler Street *(Private)*
	'Nandos', Walkergate *(Nandos)*
	'Varsity', Saddler Street *(Barracuda)*
	'Water House', North Road *(JDW)*
	'Yates's Bar', North Road *(Yates)*
	Grange Caravan Club Site *(Caravan Club)*
CP	Freeman's Quay Leisure Centre *(Private)*

Easington	Primary Care Offices, Seaside Lane (Office hrs)
Middleton-in-Teesdale	[No specific information available]
Newton Aycliffe	Newton Aycliffe Leisure Centre (Centre hrs)
Peterlee	Peterlee Leisure Centre (Centre hrs)
	'Five Quarters', Hailsham Place *(JDW)*
Seaham	Seaham Hall Car Park
	Seaham Leisure Centre (Centre hrs)
	Town Centre
	Vane Tempest Car Park
Staindrop	[No specific information available]
Stanhope	Durham Dales Visitor Centre
Stanley	Stanley Bus Station
Wearhead	by Bridge

Gateshead

Birtley	Harraton Terrace
Blaydon	The Precinct
Gateshead	Gateshead Shopping Centre *(Private)*
	'Baja Beach Club', Pipewellgate *(Private)*
	CP Chowdene Children's Centre (Centre hrs)
	CP Gateshead Central Library (Library hrs)
	CP Gateshead Civic Centre (Centre hrs)
	CP Sage Gateshead *(Private)*
Lamesley	'Ravensworth Arms' *(Private)*
Leam Lane	**CP** Gateshead @ Leam Lane (Office hrs)
Lowfell	Lowerys Lane
MetroCentre	**CP** MetroCentre, Red Mall
	Debenhams Store, Redpath Way *(Debenhams)*
	'Nandos', Garden Walk *(Nandos)*
	'Nandos', Russell Way *(Nandos)*
	'Wetherspoons', MetroCentre *(JDW)*
	Gala Bingo, Metro Retail Park *(Gala)*
Teams	**CP** Teams Children's Centre, Rose St (Centre hrs)
Whickham	'Woodmans Arms' Whickham Park *(Private)*

Hartlepool

Hartlepool	Central Library, York Road, (Library hrs)
	Place in the Park, Ward Jackson Park (10.00-16.00)
	Stockton Street Car Park (7.30-18.00)
	Town Hall Theatre Foyer (Theatre hrs)
	Hartlepool Station *(Northern Rail)*
	'King John's Tavern', South Road *(JDW)*
	'Ward Jackson', Church Square *(JDW)*
	'Yates's Bar', Victoria Road *(Yates)*
Old Hartlepool	Lighthouse
Seaton Carew	Clock Tower (M+F) (Daytime)

Middlesbrough

Middlesbrough	**CP**	Bus Station (2)
		Captain Cook Car Park
		Zetland Car Park
		Hillstreet Shopping Centre (2) *(Private)*
		The Mall Middlesbrough *(Private)*
		Middlesbrough Station *(Transpennine)*
		Debenhams Store, Newport Rd *(Debenhams)*
		'Isaac Walton', Wilson Street *(JDW)*
		'Nandos', North Ormsby Road *(Nandos)*
		'The Resolution', Newport Crescent *(JDW)*
		'The Shakespeare', Linthorpe Road *(Private)*
		'Walkabout', Corporation Road *(Private)*
		'The Welly', Albert Road *(M&B)*
	CP	James Cook University Hospital (Hospital hrs)
North Ormesby		Market Square
		'The Buccaneer', Kings Road *(M&B)*

Newcastle Upon Tyne

Benwell	West End Customer Service Centre (Centre hrs)
	'Fox & Hounds', West End *(Private)*
Byker	East End Customer Services Centre (Centre hrs)
	East End Library, Hadrian Sq (Library hrs)
	East End Pool, Foyer (Pool hrs)
	Shields Road/Edwin Street
Fenham	West Road Crematorium (Crematorium hrs)

Gosforth	Gosforth Library, Regent Farm Rd (Library hrs)
	'Andrianos', High Street *(Private)*
	'Job Bulman', St Nicholas Avenue *(JDW)*
	'Scalini's', Great North Road *(Private)*
Kenton	Kingston Park Stadium, East Stand *(N'castle Falcons)*
Newburn	Newburn Country Park (9.00-22.00)
Newcastle upon Tyne	Barrack Road, by St James Park (7.30-16.00)
	Chillingham Rd/Tosson Terrace
	CP City Library. Newbridge Street (Library hrs)
	Dean Street MSCP
	Eldon Gardens MSCP (8.00-22.00)
	Eldon Square, Sidgate (Trading hrs)
	Exhibition Park (7.30-21.00)
	Grainger Market (Market hrs)
	Haymarket, by Metro Station
	Newgate Street Car Park (Trading hrs)
	Paddy Freemans Park
	Percy Street Bus Concourse, Eldon Square
	Watergate, Quayside, by Swing Bridge
	The Gate Centre, Newgate Street *(Private)*
	Fenwicks Store, Northumberland Street *(Private)*
	Newcastle Station, Platform 4 *(East Coast)*
	'Bar 38', Lombard St. *(Private)*
	'Baron & Baroness', Times Square *(Private)*
	'Centurion', Central Station *(Private)*
	'Eye on the Tyne', Broad Chare *(Greene King)*
	'Fluid Bar', Gallowgate *(Private)*
	'Hide Bar', The Gate *(Private)*
	'Keel Row', Newgate Street *(JDW)*
	'Mile Castle', Westgate Rd/Grainger St *(JDW)*
	'Mood', The Gate *(Private)*
	'Nandos', Eldon Square *(Nandos)*
	'Nandos', Newgate Street *(Nandos)*
	'The Quayside', The Close *(JDW)*
	'Raw Hide', Newgate Street *(Private)*
	'Revolution', Collingwood Street *(Private)*
	'Union Rooms', Westgate Road *(JDW)*
	'Waterline Bar', East Quayside *(Private)*
	'The Yard', Scotswood Road *(Private)*
	'Yates's Bar', Grainger Street *(Yates)*

Metro Radio Arena, Arena Way *(Private)*
CP Eldon Square Shopping Centre *(Private)*

West Denton	Denton Park Centre (Shopping hrs) Outer West Customer Service Centre (Centre hrs)
Woolsington	'Millers', Callerton Lane Ends *(Private)*

North Tyneside

Four Lane Ends	Metro Interchange
Howden	**CP** Howden Library, Churchill Street (Library hrs)
Monkseaton	Souter Park North
Marden	'Fox Hunters', Prestongate *(Private)*
North Shields	Duke Street Fish Quay Saville Street Suez Street
Tynemouth	Front Street Long Sands North (May-Sept) Tynemouth Park
Wallsend	Forum Shopping Centre Metro Bus Station Gala Bingo, Middle Engine Lane *(Gala)* **CP** Hadrian Leisure Centre (Centre hrs)
Whitley Bay	Central Lower Promenade (May-Sept) Dukes Walk, Northern Promenade Metro Station

---

SUPPORTING THE KEY SCHEME

North Tyneside Council
Environmental Services
PO Box 113
Station Road, Killingworth
Newcastle upon Tyne
NE12 6WJ
Tel: 0845 2000 103

Park Road, by Library
South Parade
'Fire Station', York Road *(JDW)*
Old Hartley Caravan Club Site *(Caravan Club)*

Northumberland

Allendale	Market Place
Alnmouth	Alnmouth Station *(Northern Rail)*
Alnwick	The Shambles
Amble	Tourist Information Centre
Ashington	Station Road (Daytime)
	off Woodburn Road (Daytime)
	;Fox Cover;, Newbiggin Road *(Private)*
	;Rohan Kanhai', Woodhorn Road *(JDW)*
	Gala Bingo, Milburn Road *(Gala)*
Bamburgh	Bamburgh Links Car Park
	Church Street
Beadnell	Car Park (Easter-October)
Bedlington	Bower Grange, Station Road (Daytime)
	Vulcan Place
Bellingham	Main Street
Berwick-upon-Tweed	Castlegate Car Park
	Eastern Lane
	Magdelene Fields
	Woolmarket
	Berwick Station, Platform 2 *(East Coast)*
	'Leaping Salmon', Golden Square *(JDW)*
Blyth	Keel Row Shopping Centre
	Market Place
Blyth Valley Links	Fort House
	Ranch Car Park
Boulmer	Coastguard Cottage
Corbridge	Princes Street
Cramlington	Gala Bingo, Forum Way *(Gala)*
Craster	Tourist Information Centre
East Ord	Ord House Country Park *(Private)*

Etal	Castle Car Park (Easter-October) *(Parish Council)*
Haltwhistle	Westgate
Heatherslaw Mill	Car Park (M+F) (Easter-October) *(Parish Council)*
Hexham	St Mary's Wynd
	The Sele
	Tyne Green
	Wentworth Car Park
	'The Forum', Market Place *(JDW)*
Holy Island	Green Lane Car Park
Housesteads	Visitor Centre *(National Trust)*
Morpeth	Back Riggs Bus Station *(Town Council)*
	Carlisle Park *(Town Council)*
	'The Black Bull', Bridge Street *(Private)*
Newbiggin by the Sea	Promenade, by The Coble (Daytime)
Norham	off West Street *(Parish Council)*
Otterburn	Main Street
Ponteland	Thornhill Road Car Park (Daytime) *(Town Council)*
Powburn	River Breamish Caravan Club Site *(Caravan Club)*
Prudhoe	Neale Street
	South Road
Riding Mill	'Wellington Hotel', Main Road *(Private)*
Seahouses	Car Park
Seaton Sluice	Fountainhead Bank Car Park (Daytime)
	West Terrace Car Park
Spittal	Promenade Car Park
	Seaview Caravan Club Site *(Caravan Club)*
Wooler	Bus Station
Wylam	Main Road

Redcar & Cleveland

Guisborough	Fountain Street Car Park
Redcar	Coatham Enclosure (April-September)
	Esplanade West Terrace
	Locke Park
	Majuba Road Amusement Park (April-Sept)

Moore Street, off High Street
The Stray, opp. Green Lane (April-Sept)
Zetland Park, The Stray
'Plimsoll Line', High Street East *(JDW)*
'Royal Standard', West Dyke Road *(Private)*

Saltburn	**CP**	Cat Nab
		Pier (Summer)

Upsall	'Cross Keys' *(Private)*

South Tyneside

Hebburn	Hebburn Shopping Centre (Mon-Sat)
	'The Longship', Usdaw Road *(Private)*

South Shields	Coast Road, Marsden
	Laygate Roundabout
	Pier Parade (Daytime)
	Promenade, Amusement Park (Summer)
	Queen Street, by Metro Station
	Sea Road
	'The Wouldhave', Mile End Road *(JDW)*
	'Yates's Bar', Mile End Road *(Yates)*

Whitburn	Cornthwaite Park Car Park

Stockton-On-Tees

Billingham	Billingham Beck Country Park
	Cowpen Bewley Woodland Park
	Town Square

Eaglescliff	Preston Park Country Park
	Preston Park Museum (Museum hrs)

Stockton-on-Tees	High Street
	Ropner Park, Hartburn
	Wellington Square Shopping Mall
	Debenhams Store, High Street *(Debenhams)*
	'Thomas Sheraton', Bridge Road *(JDW)*

Tees Barrage	White Water Caravan Club Site *(Caravan Club)*
Teesside Leisure Park	Hollywood Bowl *(AMF)*
Thornaby	Thornaby Station *(Transpennine)*
Yarm	High Street

Sunderland

Hetton	Easington Lane, High Street
	Town Centre Car Park, Front Street
Seaburn	Seaburn Centre (Daytime)
	South Bents (Summer)
Sunderland	Harbour View, Roker Seafront
	Lower Promenade, Roker Seafront
	Park Lane Interchange
	Park Parade, Roker (Daytime)
	Southwick Green
	Central Stores, Fawcett Street *(Private)*
	Debenhams Store, The Bridges *(Debenhams)*
	'Bar Me', Low Row *(Private)*
	'Lampton Worm', Victoria Building *(JDW)*
	'Nandos', 118 High Street West *(Nandos)*
	'Old Orleans', Timber Beach Road *(Private)*
	'Varsity', Green Terrace *(Barracuda)*
	'William Jameson', Fawcett Street *(JDW)*
	'Yates's Bar', Burdon Road *(Yates)*
	Gala Bingo, Pallion New Road *(Gala)*
	Stadium of Light *(Sunderland FC)*
Washington	Concord Centre, Bus Station
	'Sir William de Wessyngton' *(JDW)*
	Gala Bingo, The Galleries *(Gala)*

CN Partions & Floors Ltd

Are pleased to support Radar

SOUTH EAST SCOTLAND

East Lothian

Athelstaneford	Main Street (Summer, 9.00-21.00)
Dirleton	Yellow Craig Caravan Club Site *(Caravan Club)*
Dunbar	Bayswell Rd (10.00-17.00, later in summer) Countess Crescent (9.00-18.00, later in summer) John Muir Country Park (9.00-18.00, later in summer) Shore Road (9.00-18.00, later in summer) Skateraw (Summer, 9.00-21.00)
East Linton	East Linton Park (9.00-18.00, later in summer)
Haddington	Neilson Park Rd. (9.00-18.00, later in summer)
Longniddry	Bents 2 (9.00-21.00 summer & weekends in winter)
Musselburgh	Shorthope Street (9.00-18.00, later in summer) **CP** Fisherrow Harbour (9.00-18.00, later in summer)
North Berwick	Quality Street (9.00-18.00, later in summer)
Port Seaton	Links Rd. (9.00-20.00 summer, 10-17.00 winter)
Preston Pans	Ayres Wynd (9.00-18.00, later in summer)
Tranent	Lindores Drive (9.00-18.00, later in summer)

Edinburgh

Drumbrae South	'Rainbow Inn', Craigmount View *(Private)* **CP** Drumbrae Leisure Centre (Centre hrs)
Edinburgh	Ardmillan Terrace, Gorgie Road Bruntsfield Canonmills Castle Terrace Car Park (10.00-20.00) Hamilton Place (10.00-18.00) Haymarket, Morrison Street (M+F) (10.00-20.00) Hope Park (10.00-18.00) Joppa, Promenade Mound, by Art Gallery Nicolson Square (10.00-22.00) Ross Band Stand, W Princes St Gdns (Summer, 8.00-20.00) St James Centre (M+F) (10.00-18.00) St John's Road (10.00-18.00)

Tollcross (10.00-20.00)
West End, W Princes Street Gdns (8.00-22.00)
Edinburgh Bus Station, Elder Street *(Private)*
Edinburgh Waverley Station *(Network Rail)*
'Alexander Graham Bell', George St *(JDW)*
'Au Bar', Shandwick Place *(Private)*
'Bar 38', George Street *(Private)*
'Black Bull', Grassmarket *(Private)*
'Browns', George Street (Private)
'Edwards', South Charlotte Street *(M&B)*
'Grape', Capital Building, St Andrews Sq *(Private)*
'Hamiltons', Hamilton Place *(Private)*
'Jongleurs', Omni Centre *(Private)*
'McCowans Brew House', Fountain Park *(Private)*
'Milnes Bar', Hanover Street *(Private)*
'Nandos', Dundee Road, Fountain Park *(Nandos)*
'Nandos', 71 Lothian Road *(Nandos)*
'Playfair', Omni Centre *(JDW)*
'Slug & Lettuce', Omni Centre *(Private)*
'Standing Order', George Street *(JDW)*
'Walkabout', Omni Centre *(Private)*

National Key Scheme Toilets

Services for Communities are responsible for Edinburgh's public toilets and operate the National Key Scheme in all our toilets with disabled access.

Edinburgh has 31 public conveniences, of which 18 have disabled access. For a list of the locations of Edinburgh's public conveniences please click on http://www.edinburgh.gov.uk/internet/City_Living/CEC_public_toilets.

For further information please contact:
0131 529 3030

•EDINBVRGH•
THE CITY OF EDINBURGH COUNCIL
SERVICE FOR COMMUNITIES

	St Christophers Backpackers, Market St *(Private)*
CP	Capability Scotland, 11 Ellersley Road *(Private)*
CP	Scottish Parliament Building (Official hrs) *(SP)*
Granton	Granton Square
	Gala Bingo, West Granton Road *(Gala)*
Leith	Taylor Gardens, Gt. Junction Street
	'Foot of the Walk', Constitution Street *(JDW)*
Meadowbank	KFC Meadowbank *(KFC)*
	Gala Bingo, Moray Park *(Gala)*
Morningside	Canaan Lane (10.00-18.00)
Newcraighall	'Cuddie Brae', off City Bypass *(Private)*
Portobello	Bath Street (10.00-20.00)
	Pipe Street
Silverknowles	Edinburgh Caravan Club Site *(Caravan Club)*
South Queensferry	High Street
	Dalmeny Station *(ScotRail)*
Wester Hailes	Westside Plaza Shopping Centre *(Private)*
	Gala Bingo, Westside Plaza *(Gala)*

Falkirk

Blackness	The Square (9.00-17.00)
Bo'ness	Register Street Car Park
	Kinneil Park, by Nursery (Park hrs)
Bonnybridge	High Street Car Park
Camelon	The Hedges, Main Street
Falkirk	Callendar Park (Park hrs)
	Glebe Street (9.00-18.00)
	Public Library, Hope Street (Library hrs)
	Callendar Square Car Park *(Private)*
	The Mall Howgate (2) *(Private)*
	Falkirk Grahamston Station *(ScotRail)*
	Falkirk High Station *(ScotRail)*
	'Carron Works', Bank Street *(JDW)*
	Gala Bingo, Kerse Lane *(Gala)*
Grangemouth	'Earl of Zetland', Bo'ness Road *(JDW)*

Larbert	Larbert Station *(ScotRail)*
	'Outside Inn', Glenbervie Business Pk *(Private)*
Polmont	Polmont Station, Booking Hall *(ScotRail)*

Midlothian

| Dalkeith | 'Blacksmiths Forge', Newmills Road *(JDW)* |
| Flotterstone Glen | Visitor Centre, A707 |

Scottish Borders

Broughton	King George VI Park
Cockburnspath	Main Street
Chirnside	Cross Hill
Coldingham Sands	Beach Front
Coldstream	Courthouse
Duns	Brierybaulk
Earlston	Main Street
Eyemouth	Harbour Road Car Park
	High Street Car Park
Galashiels	Bank Street
	Bus Station
	High Street Car Park
	'Hunters Hall', High Street *(JDW)*
Greenlaw	The Square

Scottish Borders Council

For more information on Public Facilities and Access at many attractions, why not telephone for more details before you travel?

Please telephone
01835 825111 for all enquiries

 the disability rights people

Get Caravanning
A guide to helping you explore caravanning from a disabled person's point of view.

Available from Radar's online shop
www.radar-shop.org.uk

Hawick	Common Haugh Car Park, Victoria Road Howegate, Drumlanrig Square Volunteer Park
Innerleithen	Hall Street
Jedburgh	Lothian Car Park (7.30-18.00) Tourist Information Centre
Kelso	Woodmarket/Horsemarket
Lauder	Market Place
Melrose	Abbey Street Gibson Park Caravan Club Site *(Caravan Club)*
Morebattle	Main Street
Newcastleton	Langholm Street, by Fire Station
Newton St Boswells	Main Street
Peebles	Eastgate Car Park Haylodge Park (Summer) Kingsmeadows Car Park School Brae, off High Street
St. Boswells	Main Street
St Mary's Loch	by Cafe
Selkirk	Market Square Car Park
Town Yetholm	off High Street
West Linton	Main Street, opp. Graham Institute

West Lothian

Bathgate	'James Young', Hopetoun Street *(JDW)*
Linlithgow	Linlithgow Station *(ScotRail)*
Livingston	McArthurGlen Designer Outlet *(Private)* 'Almond Bank', Almondvale Boulevard *(JDW)*

Dumfries & Galloway

Annan	Downies Wynd
Ardwell	Picnic site (Summer)
Balyett	Picnic site (Summer)
Cairnryan	Picnic site (Summer)
Carsthorn	Shore Road
Castle Douglas	Market Hill Car Park
Dalbeattie	Water Street Car Park
Drummore	Harbour Road
Dumfries	Dock Park Munchies Street Whitesands Dumfries Station, Concourse *(ScotRail)* 'Robert the Bruce', Buccleuch Street *(JDW)* Gala Bingo, Shakespeare Street *(Gala)*
Gatehouse of Fleet	High Street Car Park
Glenairle Bridge	Picnic Site, A76
Glencaple	Shore Road
Glenluce	Public Hall, Main Street (Summer) Stairhaven (Summer)
Glentrool	Stroan Bridge (Summer)

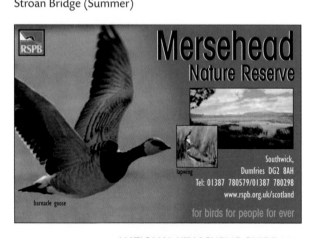

Gretna	Kirtle Place (Daytime)
Kippford	Village Hall Car Park
Kirkconnel	Main Street (M+F) (Daytime)
Kirkcudbright	Harbour Square
Langholm	Kiln Green Car Park
Lockerbie	Station Square Lockerbie Station *(ScotRail)*
Moffat	Station Park
Moniave	Ayr Road (M+F) (Daytime)
New Abbey	Car Park
Newton Stewart	Riverside Car Park Garlieston Caravan Club Site *(Caravan Club)*
Palnure	Kirroughtree Visitor Centre *(Forest Enterprise)*
Penpont	Marrburn Road Car Park (M+F) (Daytime)
Port Logan	Fish Pond Car Park New England Bay Caravan Club Site *(Caravan Club)*
Portpatrick	Harbour
Port William	Village Square
Sandhead	Main Street
Sanquhar	South Lochan (M+F) (Daytime)
Southerness	Car Park, Shore Road
Stranraer	Agnew Park Pavilion (Daytime) Hanover Square Car Park Sea Front Stair Park (Summer) Stranraer Station, Car Park *(ScotRail)*
Thornhill	St Cutherberts Walk (M+F) (Daytime)
Wanlockhead	Lead Mining Museum (Summer)
Whithorn	Bruce Street (Daytime)
Wigtown	High Vennel

East Ayrshire

Cumnock	Glaisnock Shopping Centre Cumnock Town Hall (Booking hrs)
Kilmarnock	Burns Mall Shopping Centre Dick Institute Library & Gallery (Library hrs) Kilmarnock Station, Concourse *(ScotRail)* 'Wheatsheaf Inn', Portland Street *(JDW)* Gala Bingo, Portland Street *(Gala)*
Mauchline	Loudoun Street

East Dunbartonshire

Bearsden	Bearsden Cross
Bishopbriggs	'Eagle Lodge', Hilton Road *(Private)*
Clachan of Campsie	Recreational Area
Kirkintilloch	Southbank Road 'Kirky Puffer', Townhead *(Private)*
Lenzie	Lenzie Station *(ScotRail)*
Milngavie	Mugdock Road 'Cross Keys', Station Road *(Private)* Milngavie Station *(ScotRail)*

East Renfrewshire

Barrhead	Main Street
Busby	'White Cart', East Kilbride Road *(Private)*
Eaglesham	Eaglesham Pavilion, Gilmour Street
Giffnock	Rouken Glen Park, Car Park
Mearns	The Avenue Shopping Centre *(Private)*

Glasgow

Darnley	Gala Bingo, Woodneuk Road *(Gala)*
Drumchapel	Shopping Centre Sainsbury's Store, Allerdyce Drive *(Sainsbury)*
Glasgow	Collins Street St Vincent Street, St Vincent Place Stevenson Street West Campbell Street

Buchanan Galleries *(Private)*
Princes Square, Buchanan St *(Private)*
St Enoch Shopping Centre (4) *(Private)*
Debenhams Store, Argyle St *(Debenhams)*
Buchanan Bus Station (2) *(SPT)*
Charing Cross Station *(ScotRail)*
Glasgow Central Station *(Network Rail)* (2)
Glasgow Queen Street Station *(ScotRail)*
'All Bar One', St Vincent St *(M&B)*
'The Arches', Argyle Street *(Private)*
'Bar Censsa', West George Street *(Private)*
'Barrachnie Inn', Glasgow Rd, Garrowhill *(Private)*
'Buffalo Joes', Hope Street *(Private)*
'Central Bar', Central Station *(Private)*
'Counting House', St Vincents Place *(JDW)*
'Crystal Palace', Jamaica Street *(JDW)*
'Edward Wylie', Bothwell Street **(JDW)**
'Edwards', West George Street *(M&B)*
'Esquire House', Great Western Rd *(JDW)*
'Frankenstein 1818', West George St *(Private)*
'Hengler's Circus', Sauchihall Street *(JDW)*

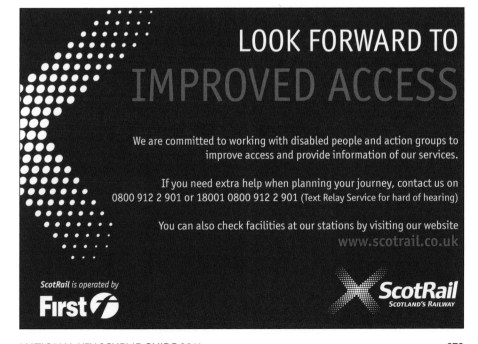

'Jongleurs', Renfrew Street *(Private)*
'Lakota', West George Street *(Private)*
'Mojama', Sauchiehall Street *(Private)*
  'Nandos', Glasgow Fort Shopping Centre *(Nandos)*
'Nandos', The Quay, West Paisley Rd *(Nandos)*
'Nandos', St Enochs Centre *(Nandos)*
'Nandos', Silverburn Shopping Centre *(Nandos)*
'O'Neills', Albion Street *(M&B)*
'Sauciehaugh', Sauchiehall Street *(Private)*
'Sir John Moore', Argyle Street *(JDW)*
'Sir John Stirling Maxwell', Kilmarnock Rd *(JDW)*
'Society Room', West George Street *(JDW)*
'Walkabout', Renfield Street *(Private)*
'Yates's Bar', Sauchiehall Street *(Yates)*
'Yates's Bar', West George Street *(Yates)*
Glasgow Caledonian University (7) *(University)*
O2 Academy, Eglinton Street *(Private)*
Scottish Exhibition & Conference Centre *(Private)*

Mount Florida	Langside College, Business School *(College)*
	Langside College, LITE House *(College)*
Parkhead	Forge Shopping Centre, Gallowgate *(Private)*
Partick	Partick Interchange *(SPT)* [Planned]
	Glasgow University Union *(University)*
	Queen Margaret Union *(University)*
Possil Park	Gala Bingo, Hawthorn Street *(Gala)*

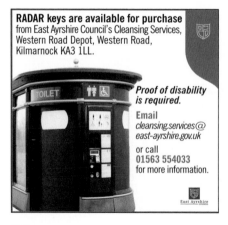
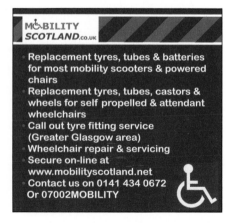

Inverclyde

Gourock	Albert Road (Daytime)
	Shore Street (Daytime)
	Gourock Station *(ScotRail)*
Greenock	Campbell Street (Daytime)
	Hunters Place
	Kilblain Street (Daytime)
	Greenock Central Station *(ScotRail)*
	'James Watt', Cathcart Street *(JDW)*
Inverkip	Greenock Road (Daytime)
Port Glasgow	Coronation Park (Daytime)
	Port Glasgow Station *(ScotRail)*
Wemyss Bay	Wemyss Bay Station *(ScotRail)*

North Ayrshire

Ardrossan	North Crescent Road (9.00-17.00)
Irvine	East Road (9.00-18.00)
	Low Green Road (9.00-14.00, later in summer)
	Shorehead (Summer, daytime)
	Irvine Station *(ScotRail)*
	Gala Bingo, Townhead *(Gala)*
Isle of Arran	Blackwaterfoot, Harbour
	Brodick, Public Green (Daytime in winter)
	Lamlash, Shore Road
	Whiting Bay, Shore Road
Kilwinning	Abbey Green
	Kilwinning Station *(ScotRail)*
Largs	Pierhead (Daytime)
	Largs Station *(ScotRail)*
Saltcoats	The Braes (9.30-20.00, later in summer)
	Melbourne Gardens (Apr-Sept 9.30-20.00)
	'The Salt Cot', Hamilton Street *(JDW)*
Stevenston	Alexander Place/Main Street
	Stevenston Shore (Summer 12.00-18.00)

North Lanarkshire

Airdrie	Town Centre 'Robert Hamilton', Bank Street *(JDW)*
Bellshill	North Road 'Avondale Bar/Lily Restaurant' *(Private)* **CP** Sir Matt Busby Sports Centre (Centre hrs)
Coatbridge	Main Street 'The Vulcan', Main Street *(JDW)* **CP** Summerlee Museum of Scottish Industrial Life
Croy	Croy Station, Ticket Office *(ScotRail)*
Cumbernauld	Tay Walk (Shopping hrs) *(Private)* Teviot Walk (Shopping hrs) *(Private)* Cumbernauld Station *(ScotRail)* **CP** Tryst Sports Complex (Centre hrs)
Kilsyth	King Street
Moodiesburn	**CP** Pivot Community Education Centre (Centre hrs)
Motherwell	Brandon Parade South Motherwell Station *(ScotRail)*

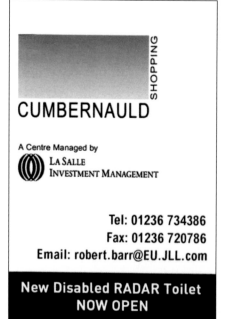

SHOPPING

CUMBERNAULD

A Centre Managed by

LA SALLE INVESTMENT MANAGEMENT

Tel: 01236 734386
Fax: 01236 720786
Email: robert.barr@EU.JLL.com

New Disabled RADAR Toilet NOW OPEN

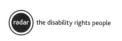

radar the disability rights people

Doing Work Differently

Part of our 'Doing Life Differently' series,
this toolkit explores practical solutions to real
questions related to work.

Available from Radar's online shop
www.radar-shop.org.uk

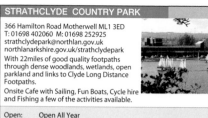

STRATHCLYDE COUNTRY PARK

366 Hamilton Road Motherwell ML1 3ED
T: 01698 402060 M: 01698 252925
strathclydepark@northlan.gov.uk
northlanarkshire.gov.uk/strathclydepark
With 22miles of good quality footpaths
through dense woodlands, wetlands, open
parkland and links to Clyde Long Distance
Footpaths.
Onsite Cafe with Sailing, Fun Boats, Cycle hire
and Fishing a few of the activities available.

Open: Open All Year
            Various times during winter and summer months more
            details on web site.
Admission: Free

	'Brandon Works', Merry Street *(JDW)*
CP	Isa Community Centre (Centre hrs)
Muirhead	'Muirhead Hotel' *(Private)*
Shotts	**CP** Shotts Community Centre
Uddingstone	**CP** Viewpark Community Centre
Wishaw	Kenilworth Avenue
	CP Wishaw Library
	'Wishaw Malt', Kirk Road *(JDW)*

Renfrewshire

Braehead	**CP** Braehead Shopping Centre *(Private)*
	'Lord of the Isles', Xscape *(JDW)*
	'Nandos', Xscape *(Nandos)*
	BowlPlex, Xscape *(BowlPlex)*
Paisley	Barshaw Park
	Paisley Gilmour Street Station *(ScotRail)*
	'Last Post', County Square *(JDW)*
	Gala Bingo, Phoenix Retail Park *(Gala)*
Renfrew	Inchinnan Road

South Ayrshire

Ayr	Arthur Street (10.00-19.00)
	Blackburn Car Park, Sea Front (Summer 10.00-19.00)
	Pavilion, Esplanade (M+F) (10.00-19.00)
	Ayr Station, Concourse *(ScotRail)*
	'West Kirk', Sandgate *(JDW)*
	Craigie Gardens Caravan Club Site *(Caravan Club)*
Ballintrae	Forelands
Dunure	Kennedy Park (Summer 10.00-19.00)
Girvan	Ainslie Car Park
	Flushes Car Park
	Girvan Station *(ScotRail)*
Maidens	Harbour
Prestwick	Boydfield Gardens
	Links Road (Summer & weekends in winter) *(Private)*
	Prestwick Town Station *(ScotRail)*
Prestwick Airport	Prestwick Airport Station *(ScotRail)*

Troon	Church Street (10.00-19.00)
	Fullarton Estate (8.00-20.00)
	St Meddans Street Car Park (10.00-19.00)
	Troon Station *(ScotRail)*

South Lanarkshire

Biggar	Main Street (Daytime)
Carluke	Carnwath Road (Daytime)
	CP Carluke Lifestyles (Centre hrs)
Carnwath	Main Street
Carstairs	Carstairs Station *(ScotRail)*
Crossford	Lanark Road (Daytime)
East Kilbride	Greenhills Shopping Centre
	Maxwell Drive
	CP Murray Owen Centre, Liddell Grove
	Plaza Centre, Mall (Shopping hrs)
	St Leonards Shopping Centre (8.00-20.00)
	'Peel Park', Eaglesham Road *(Private)*
Forth	Main Street (Daytime)
Hamilton	Bus Station, Brandon House (Daytime)
	CP Lifestyles Leisure Centre (Centre hrs)
Kirkfieldbank	Riverside Road
Lanark	Horsemarket (Daytime)
	'Clydesdale Inn', Bloomgate *(JDW)*
Larkhall	King Street
Law	Station Road
Leadhills	Main Street
Rutherglen	Arcade
	King Street
	CP Lifestyles Leisure Centre (Centre hrs)
Stonehouse	King Street
Strathaven	Green Street

West Dunbartonshire

Alexandria	Main StreetOvertoun Road
	Leven Vale Pool (Pool hrs)
Balloch	Old Balloch Station, by TIC
Clydebank	**CP** The Playdrome, Abbotsford Road (Centre hrs)
	Clyde Shopping Centre *(Private)*
	In Shops, Syvania Road South *(Private)*
	'KFC', Livingstone Street *(KFC)*
	Gala Bingo, Kilbowie Retail Park *(Gala)*
Dumbarton	Riverside Lane (2)
	CP Dumbarton Disability Resource Centre

Aberdeen City

Aberdeen		Central Library (Library hrs)
		Skene Street/Summer Street
		Stonehaven Road, A90 Lay-by
		Debenhams Store, Trinity Centre *(Debenhams)*
		Aberdeen Station, Concourse *(ScotRail)*
		'Archibald Simpson', Castle Street *(JDW)*
		'Beluga', Union Street *(Private)*
		'Cocket Hat', North Anderson Drive *(Private)*
		'J G Ross Coffee Shop', King St *(Private)*
		'Justice Mill', Union Street *(JDW)*
		'Nandos', Union Square *(Nandos)*
		'Slains Castle', Belmont Street *(Private)*
		Gala Bingo, King Street *(Gala)*
		Lynx Ice Centre (Centre hrs)
Cults		North Deeside Road, by Library
Kincorth	**CP**	Kincorth Sports Centre, Corthan Crescent (Centre hrs)
Mastrick		Sheddocksley Sports Centre (Centre hrs)
Peterculter		North Deeside Road, by restaurant

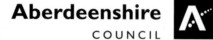

Aberdeenshire

COUNCIL

For more information on public facilities and access to many attractions, why not telephone for more details before you travel.

Please telephone for all enquiries:

08456 08 1207

Aberdeenshire

Aberchider	Market Street
Aboyne	Ballater Road
Alford	Car Park
Auchenblae	Mackenzie Avenue
Auchnagatt	Martin Terrace *(Community Council)*
Ballater	The Square
Balmedie	The Haughs (Summer, daytime)
Banchory	Bellfield Car Park
	Silverbank Caravan Club Site *(Caravan Club)*
Banff	Duff House Grounds
	Marina (8.00-17.00)
	St Mary's Car Park
	Harbour (June-Aug) *(Community Council)*
Bellabeg	Strathdon
Bennachie	Rowan Tree Car Park (April-October)
Boddam	Harbour Street
Braemar	Ballnellan Road
	Invercauld Caravan Club Site *(Caravan Club)*
Cornhill	Mid Street
Crathie	Car Park (April-October)
Crimond	Logie Drive
Ellon	Market Street
Fordyce	East Church Street
Fraserburgh	Castle Street
	Interpretive Centre
	Bus Station, Hanover Street *(Private)*
Fyvie	Cummiestown Road
Gardenstown	The Harbour
Gourdon	Boath Park
Hatton	Station Road
Huntly	Castle Street
	Market Muir

Inverallochy	Allochy Road
Inverurie	Station Road
Johnshaven	Fore Street
Maud	Station Road
Mintlaw	Aden Country Park, Coach House (Park hrs)
	Aden Country Park, Bottom Car Park (Summer)
	Aden Country Park Top Car Park (Summer)
	The Square
New Byth	Playing Fields
New Pitsligo	High Street/Market Place
Oldmeldrum	Urquhart Road
Peterhead	Drummers Corner/Tolbooth
	'Cross Keys', Back Street *(JDW)*
	Gala Bingo, Marischal Street *(Gala)*
Port Elphinstone	Port Road
Portsoy	Short Street
Potarch	Potarch Green
Rosehearty	Union Street
Stonehaven	Harbour
	Margaret Street
Strichen	Bridge Street
Stuartfield	Knock Field (April-October)
Tarves	Pleasure Park, Tolquhon Avenue

Turriff	High Street
Westhill	Shopping Centre
	'Shepherds Rest', Arnhall Business Pk. *(Private)*

Angus

Arbroath	Hamilton Green
	Harbour Visitor Centre
	Market Place
	Ness-Victoria Park
	Tennis Courts (April-October)
	Arbroath Station *(ScotRail)*
	'Corn Exchange', Market Place *(JDW)*
	Gala Bingo, High Street *(Gala)*
	CP Lochlands Adult Resource Centre (Centre hrs)
Auchmithie	Fountain Square
Brechin	Church Street
Carnoustie	Carnoustie House Parks (Events only)
	Ferrier Street
Edzell	The Muir
Forfar	Buttermarket
	Lochside Caravan Club Site *(Caravan Club)*
	CP Lilybank Resource Centre (Centre hrs)
Kirriemuir	**CP** Websters Sports Centre (Centre hrs)
Monifieth	Riverview Drive, Play Area (April-Sept)
Montrose	Trail Pavilion
	Town Buildings
	Montrose Station *(ScotRail)*
	Gala Bingo, Hume Street *(Gala)*
	CP Rosehill Resource Centre (Centre hrs)

Clackmannanshire

Alloa	**CP** Alloa Leisure Bowl (Centre hrs)

Dundee

Broughty Ferry	**CP**	Beach, Windmill Gardens (9.00-18.00) Queen Street Car Park 'Bell Tree', Panmurefield Road *(Private)*
Dundee		Hilltown McManus Galleries (Museum hrs) Seagate Bus Station (Daytime) Tayside House (Office hrs) Wellgate Library (Library hrs) Debenhams Store, Overgate *(Debenhams)* Dundee Station *(ScotRail)* 'The Capitol', Seagate *(JDW)* 'Counting House', Reform Street *(JDW)* 'Outside Inn', Camperdown Park *(Private)* Gala Bingo, The Stack Leisure Park *(Gala)*
	CP	Dallhouse Building, Old Hawkhill *(Dundee University)*
	CP	Ninewells Hospital (Hospital hrs)
	CP	Pamis, Springfield House, Dundee University *(Private)*
	CP	White Top Centre (Centre hrs)
Lochee		Aimer Square Car Park

Fife

Aberdour		Aberdour Station *(ScotRail)*
Burntisland		Links Place (8.30-19.00, later in Summer)
Cowdenbeath		Cowdenbeath Station *(ScotRail)*
Cupar		Bonnygate Car Park Cupar Station *(ScotRail)*
Dunfermline		Dunfermline Town Station *(ScotRail)* 'Nandos', Fife Leisure Park *(Nandos)* Bowlplex, Fife Leisure Park *(Bowlplex)*
	CP	Tuloch Leisure Centre (Centre hrs)
	CP	Lynebank Wheelchair Clinic (Centre hrs)
Elie		Pavilion Café, Golf Course Lane *(Private)*
Glenrothes		Bus Station *(Private)* Kingdom Shopping Centre (2) *(Private)* 'Golden Acorn', North Street *(JDW)*
	CP	Fife Inst. of Physical & Recreational Education (Centre hrs)

Inverkeithing	Inverkeithing Station *(ScotRail)*
	'Burgh Arms', High Street *(Private)*
Kinghorn	Kinghorn Station *(ScotRail)*
Kirkcaldy	Esplanade (8.30-19.00)
	Kirkcaldy Station *(ScotRail)*
	William Hill, Dunearn Drive *(Private)*
	'Robert Nairn', Kirk Wynd *(JDW)*
Leuchars	Leuchars Station *(ScotRail)*
Leven	Promenade (10.00-16.00, later in summer)
	Bus Station, Branch Street *(Private)*
CP	Levenmouth Swimming Pool (Pool hrs)
Markinch	Markinch Station *(Scotrail)*
	Balbirnie Park Caravan Club Site *(Caravan Club)*
Pittenweem	The Harbour (Daytime)
St Andrews	Bruce Embankment (Daytime)
St Monans	Hope Place (Daytime)
Tayport	The Harbour

Perth & Kinross

Auchterarder	Crown Wynd Car Park
Blair Atholl	Village Hall Car Park
Blairgowrie	Wellmeadow
Comrie	Dalginross
Crieff	James Square
Dunkeld	North Car Park
Perth	A K Bell Library, York Place (Library hrs)
	Bus Station, Leonard Street
	Marshall Place (8.00-18.00)
	Ropemakers Close (8.30-18.00)
	St Johns Shopping Centre *(Private)*
	Perth Station, Entrance Hall *(ScotRail)*
	'Capital Asset', Tay Street *(JDW)*
CP	Bells Sports Centre (Centre hrs)
Pitlochry	West Lane (9.00-18.00)
	Pitlochry Station *(ScotRail)*

St Fillans	Main Street
Turfhills M90	Kinross Services, J6 M90 *(Moto)*

Stirling

Callander	South Church Street
	Station Road
Crianlarich	Glenfalloch Road
Dunblane	Dunblane Station, Platform 1 *(ScotRail)*
Killin	Maragowan Caravan Club Site *(Caravan Club)*
Lochearnhead	Crieff Road
Stirling	Bus Station *(Private)*
	Stirling Station, Platform 2 *(ScotRail)*
	Debenhams Store, Thistle Centre *(Debenhams)*
	'Nandos', Forthside *(Nandos)*
	Stirling Bowl, Forth Street *(AMF)*
CP	Riverbank Resource Centre (Centre hrs)

HIGHLANDS & ISLANDS

Argyll & Bute

Ardrishaig	Car Park (8.00-17.00, later in summer)
Campbeltown	Bolgam Street, off Main Street (8.00-18.00)
	Pensioners Row (9.30-17.00)
Dunoon	Moir Street (8.00-22.00)
Helensburgh	Kidston Park, The Pier (9.00-14.00, later in summer)
Innellan	Shore Road, Sandy Beach (Summer)
Inveraray	The Pier (7.00-20.30, later in summer)
Isle of Bute	Ettrick Bay (April-Sept 10.00-19.00)
	Port Bannatyne
	Rothsey Pier
Isle of Gigha	Ferry Car Park, Ardminish
Isle of Islay	Bowmore, School Street
	Feolin
	Port Askaig, CalMac Building

Best wishes to Radar from

Argyll and Bute Council
OPERATIONAL SERVICES DEPARTMENT

Roads and Amenity Services
1a Manse Brae
Lochgilphead
PA31 8RD

Tel: 01546 604 614

	Port Ellen, Charlotte Street
	Portnahaven
Isle of Mull	Craignure
	Fionnphort
	Tobermory *(Harbour Assn)*
Kilcreggan	Pier (9.00-16.00, later in summer)
Killegruer	Glenbarr Caravan Site
Lochgilphead	Lochnell St (7,00-17.00, later in summer)
Loch Lomond	Firkin Point (8.00-16.00, later in summer)
Luss	Car Park (8.00-16.00, later in summer)
Oban	Oban Station *(ScotRail)*
Rhu	Main Road (9.00-16.00, later in summer)
Sandbank	Main Road (8.00-20.00)
Tarbert	Harbour Street (7.00-18.00, later in summer)
Tayinloan	Village Centre
Taynuilt	School Road

Highland

Achiltibuie	North of Village
Achnasheen	Achnasheen Station *(ScotRail)*
Applecross	Shore Street
Arisaig	by village shop
Ardgay	[No specific information available] (Summer only)
Aviemore	Main Street
Beauly	High Street (M+F)
Bettyhill	Car Park, A836
Bonar Bridge	Picnic Site
Brora	Dalcham Caravan Club Site *(Caravan Club)*
Carrbridge	Car Park
Clachtoll	Beach
Corran	by Ferry
Cromarty	Allan Square

Culloden	Culloden Moor Caravan Club Site *(Caravan Club)*
Daviot Wood	A9 Northbound, by Information Centre
Dingwall	Tulloch Street
Dores	Dores Inn
Drumbeg	Car Park
Drumnadrochit	Tourist Information Centre Car Park
Dunbeath	Harbour
Dunnet Bay	Beach
Fort Augustus	A82, by Tourist Information Centre
Fort William	Viewforth Car Park Fort William Station *(ScotRail)*
Gairloch	Community Centre (M+F) (Centre hrs) Harbour Road
Golspie	Car Park off Main Street **CP** Sutherland Swimming Pool (Pool hrs)
Glencoe	Car Park opp. hotel
Grantown	High Street (April-Oct) Burnfield
Invergordon	King Street
Invermoriston	Glenmoriston Millennium Hall
Inverness	Castle Wynd Mealmarket Close Inverness Station *(ScotRail)* 'The Fluke', Culcabock Road *(Private)* 'Kings Highway', Church Street *(JDW)*
Isle of Skye	Ardvasar, Village Hall Broadford, opp. Visitor Car Park Carbost, opp. The Distillery Dunvegan, Visitor Car Park Kilmuir, by Thatched Museum Portree, Camanachd Square Portree, The Green Uig, Visitor Car Park **CP** Portree, The Fingal Centre (Pool hrs)
John O'Groats	Car Park

Keiss	Main Street
Kinlochewe	Slioch Terrace
	Kinlochewe Caravan Club Site *(Caravan Club)*
Kinlochleven	nr. Ice Factor
Kyle of Lochalsh	Car Park
	Kyle of Lochalsh Station *(ScotRail)*
Lairg	Main Street
Lochcarron	by Village Hall
Lochinver	Main Street
Mallaig	East Bay Car Park
	Mallaig Station *(ScotRail)*
Muir of Ord	Seaforth Road
Nairn	Court House Lane
	East Beach, Car Park
	Harbour Street
	The Links, West Beach
	Mill Road
North Kessock	Picnic Area, A9 Northbound (Daytime)
	Picnic Area, A9 Southbound (Daytime)
Onich	Bunree Caravan Club Site *(Caravan Club)*
Portmahomack	Main Street (April-October)
Rogie Falls	Car Park, A835 (April-October)
Rosemarkie	Mill Road
Shiel Bridge	Morvich Caravan Club Site *(Caravan Club)*
Silver Bridge	Car Park, A835
Smoo	Smoo Cave
Strathpeffer	The Square (April-October)
Tain	Rose Garden, off High Street (2)
Tarbet, Sutherland	Tarbet Pier
Thurso	Harbour
	Tanyard, Riverside Road
Ullapool	West Argyle Street (M+F)
Wick	Whitechapel Road

Wick Station *(ScotRail)*
'Alexander Blain', Market Place *(JDW)*

Moray

Aberlour	Alice Littler Park (8.00-16.00, later in summer)
Buckie	Fish Market (8.00-16.00, later in summer)
	Newlands Lane Car Park (8.00-17.00, later in summer)
	CP Burney Day Centre (Centre hrs)
Burghhead	Harbour (8.00-16.00, later in summer)
Craigellachie	Victoria Road, A95 *(Community Council)*
Cullen	Cullen Harbour (April-October 8.00-20.00)
	The Square (8.00-16.00, later in summer)
Dufftown	Albert Place Car Park (8.00-16.00, later in summer)
Elgin	Elgin Library (Library hrs)
	Cooper Park (April-Oct, 8.00-20.00)
	Elgin Station *(ScotRail)*
	Tesco Store, Lossie Green *(Tesco)*
	'Muckle Cross', High Street *(JDW)*
	CP Cedarwood Day Service (Centre hrs)
Findhorn	The Beach, Middle Block (M+F)
	The Beach, West Block (M+F)
Findochty	Edindoune Shore (8.00-16.00, later in summer)
Forres	Grant Park (April-Oct, 8.00-20.00)
	The Leys (9.00-17.00, later in summer)
	Forres Station *(ScotRail)*
Garmouth	Playing Field (April-October)
Hopeman	Harbour (8.00-16.00, later in summer)
Keith	Regent Square (8.00-16.00, later in summer)
	Reidhaven (8.00-16.00, later in summer) (M+F)
	Keith Station *(ScotRail)*
Lossiemouth	Esplanade (8.00-16.00, later in summer) (M+F)
	Station Park (8.00-16.00, later in summer)
Portknockie	Harbour (April-Oct, 8.00-20.00)
Rothes	New Street (8.00-16.00, later in summer) (M+F)
Tomintoul	Back Lane (8.00-16.00, later in summer)

Orkney Islands

Deerness	Community Hall *(Community Council)*
Evie	Aikerness
	Tingwall Pier Waiting Room
Finstown	Maitland Place
Kirkwall	Peedie Sea Boat Store, Pickaquoy Road
	CP Kirkwall Travel Centre (Centre hrs)
	Shapinsay Ferry Terminal (Terminal hrs)
	Shore Street
	Scapa Beach
Orphir	Waulkmill
Sanday	Kettletoft Pier Waiting Room
Sandwick	Bay of Skaill
South Ronaldsay	Sands O'Wright
	4th Barrier
Stromness	Ferry Road
	Warbeth Beach
Stronsay	Whitehall Pier

Western Isles Council

For more information on Public Facilities and Access at many attractions, why not telephone for more details before you travel?

Please telephone for all enquiries:

0845 600 7090

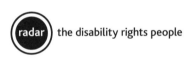 **radar** the disability rights people

Gabh ballrachd de Radar

Lìonra de dhaoine aig a bheil ùidhean co-ionann agus airson fios air saoghal nan daoine ciorramach.

www.radar.org.uk

Shetland Islands

Lerwick	**CP**	Harbour House
		The Viking Bus Station
Scalloway		Burn Beach Car Park (8.00-21.00)

Western Isles

Stornoway	Percival Square, opp. Tourist Information Centre

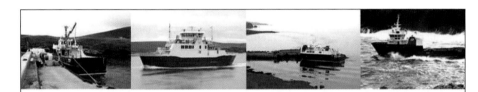

Inter Island Ferry Service - Gateway to the isles

Shetland Islands Council runs a network of inter-island ferries that makes it quick and easy to travel to and from the isles, with or without a vehicle and all for very reasonable fares. With 190 sailings per day, it is just like hopping on a bus!

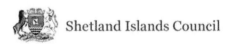 Shetland Islands Council

01595 744 252   www.shetland.gov.uk/ferries

Isle Of Anglesey

Aberffraw	Llys Llywelyn (Summer)
Amlwch	Lon Goch
Beaumaris	by Library
Benllech	Beach Car Park (Summer)
	Square Car Park
Brynsiencyn	Car Park (Summer)
Cemaes	Beach Car Park
	High Street
Church Bay	Beach Car Park (Summer)
Holyhead	Breakwater Park (Summer)
	Newry Beach
	Porth Dafarch (Summer)
	South Stack (Summer)
	Swift Square
	Holyhead Ferry Terminal *(Stena)*
Llanddona	Beach (Summer)
Llaneilian	Beach (Summer)
Llanfairpwll	Car Park, by Post Office
Llangefni	Lon y Felin
Llannerch-y-Medd	High Street
Menai Bridge	Bowling Green/Beach Road (Summer)
	Library
	Pier
CP	Pilipalas Nature World *(Private)*
Newborough	Beach Road Car Park (Summer)
Penrhos	Nature Reserve Beach (Summer)
	Penrhos Caravan Club Site *(Caravan Club)*
Red Wharf Bay	[No specific information available] (Summer)
Rhoscolyn	Beach Car Park (Summer)
Rhosneigr	Library Car Park

Traeth Bychan	Car Park (Summer)
Trearddur Bay	Beach Car Park (Summer)
Valley	Council Car Park

Conwy

Abergele	Beefield, Car Park
	Water Street
Betwys-y-Coed	Pont-y-Pair Car Park
	Station Road Car Park
Cerrigydrudion	Tan Llan, off A55
Colwyn Bay	The Close
	Douglas Road Car Park
	Eiras Park
	Eiras Park Coach Park
	Ivy Street
	Lansdowne Road Car Park
	Promenade, Central
	Promenade, Dingle (April-September)
	Colwyn Bay Station *(Arriva Wales)*
	'Picture House', Princes Drive *(JDW)*

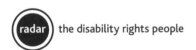 the disability rights people

Dewch i fod yn aelod o Radar

Rhwydweithio gyda phobl o'r un anian a chadw i fyny â newyddion sector anabledd.

www.radar.org.uk

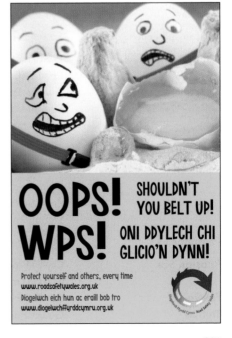

OOPS! SHOULDN'T YOU BELT UP!
WPS! ONI DDYLECH CHI GLICIO'N DYNN!

Protect yourself and others, every time
www.roadsafetywales.org.uk
Diogelwch eich hun ac eraill bob tro
www.diogelwchffyrddcymru.org.uk

Conwy	Bodlondeb (April-September)
	Morfa Bach Car Park (April-September)
	The Quay
	Castle Visitor Centre *(Cadw)*
Deganwy	Level Crossing
Dolwyddelan	by Post Office
Kinmel Bay	The Square, Foryd Road
Llanddulas	Station Road (April-September)
Llandudno	George Street
	Great Orme Visitor Centre (April-September)
	Happy Valley Road
	Llanrhos Cemetery
	Mostyn Broadway Coach Park
	North Shore, nr. Paddling Pool
	Llandudno Station *(Arriva Wales)*
	Dale Park Café, West Shore *(Private)*
	'The Palladium', Gloddaeth Street *(JDW)*
Llandudno Junction	Osborne Road Car Park, off A55
	Llandudno Junction Station *(Arriva Wales)*
CP	Welsh Assembly Government.Office *(WA)*
Llanelian	by Recreation Field (April-September)
Llanfair Talhaearn	School Lane, off A548
Llanfairfechan	Promenade, Car Park
	Rhandir Cemetery
Llanrwst	Gwydyr Park (April-September)
	Plas-yn-Dre
	Watling Street
Llansannan	Canol y Llan
Penmaenmawr	Fernbrook Road Car Park, off A55
	Promenade by Subway *(April-September)*
	Promenade, West End *(April-September)*
	Station Road Car Park
Pentrefoelas	Monument, off A55
Rhos-on-Sea	Cayley Promenade
	Marine Drive (April-September)
Towyn	Sandbank Road
Trefriw	Gower Road

Denbighshire

Corwen	Rug Chapel *(Cadw)*
Denbigh	Rosemary Lane
Llangollen	Market Street
Loggerheads	Country Park (Park hrs)
Prestatyn	Barkby Beach
	Bus Station, Ffordd Pendyffryn
	Council Offices, Nant Hall Road (Office hrs)
	The Nova, Central Beach
	Prestatyn Station *(Arriva Wales)* [2010/11]
Rhuddlan	Princes Road (dawn-dusk)
Rhyl	Coromation Gardens (Park hrs)
	Events Arena (Daytime)
	Old Golf Road (Daytime)
	Railway Station (Daytime)
	Town Hall
	Rhyl Station *(Arriva Wales)*
	'Sussex', Sussex Street *(JDW)*
Ruthin	Market Street
St Asaph	High Street, nr. Bridge (Daytime)

Flintshire

Caerwys	Drovers Lane
Cilcain	Village Community Centre
Connah's Quay	Fron Road
Flint	Flint Station *(Arriva Wales)*
Holywell	Somerfield Car Park
	Tower Gardens Car Park
Mold	Bus Station
	Daniel Owen Centre (Mon-Sat 8.00-18.00)
	New Street Car Park
	'Gold Cape', Wrexham Street *(JDW)*
Saltney	High Street
Shotton	Alexander Street
	'Central Hotel', Chester Road West *(JDW)*

Gwynedd

Aberdaron	The Beach (Easter-Oct, daytime)
Aberdyfi	The Quay
Abersoch	Golf Road (Easter-Oct) The Harbour (Easter-Oct)
Bala	The Green Plassey Street
Bangor	Glanrafon (Daytime) Tan y Fynwent (Daytime) Bangor Station *(Arriva Wales)* 'Black Bull Inn', High Street *(JDW)* 'Varsity', High Street *(Barracuda)*
Barmouth/Abermaw	Llys Cambrian, nr Station (Daytime) The Quay (Daytime) North Parade (Easter-Oct, daytime) Barmouth Station *(Arriva Wales)*
Beddgelert	Village Ty Isaf *(National Trust)*

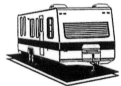

Blaenau Ffestiniog	Diffwys Coed-y-Llwyn Caravan Club Site *(Caravan Club)*
Caernarfon	Castle Hill (Daytime) by Empire (Daytime) Penllyn Car Park (Daytime) 'Tafarn y Porth', Eastgate Street *(JDW)*
Criccieth	Car Park (Daytime) Esplanade (Easter-Oct, daytime) Marine (Easter-Oct, daytime) Criccieth Castle *(Cadw)*
Dinas Dinlle	by The Marine (Daytime)
Dolgellau	Marian Mawr Car Park
Fairbourne/Y Friog	Penrhyn Drive South
Harlech	Bron y Graig by Castle (Easter-September)
Llanberis	Ger y Llyn (Daytime) Maes Padarn (Daytime) Y Glyn (M+F) (Easter-Sept, daytime)
Llandanwg	The Beach
Llithfaen	Village
Machroes	by Beach (Easter-Oct, daytime)
Maentwrog	by Oakeley Arms
Morfa Bychan	Beach Entrance (Easter-Oct)
Mynytho	Chwarel Foel Gron (Easter-Oct)
Nefyn	Cefn Twr (Daytime)
Penrhyndeudraeth	Car Park (Daytime)
Porthmadog	Public Park (Daytime)
Pwllheli	Penlan (Daytime) South Beach (Daytime) Y Maes/The Square (Daytime) West End (Daytime)
Trawsfynydd	Car Park
Trefor	Y Traeth/Beach (Easter-Sept, daytime)
Tudweiliog	Village (Apr-Oct)

Tywyn	by Cinema
	Recreation Ground
Y Felinheli	Beach Road

Wrexham

Cefn-Mawr	Ty-Mawr Country Park (Park hrs)
Chirk	Colliery Road Car Park
	Lady Margaret's Park Caravan Club Site *(Caravan Club)*
Coedpoeth	High Street Car Park
Erddig	Country Park *(National Trust)*
Holt	Cross Street *(Community Council)*
Overton	School Street Car Park *(Community Council)*
Rhosllanerchrugog	Market Street
Rossett	The Green, Chester Road *(Community Council)*
Trevor	Canal Basin Car Park
Wrexham	Henblas Street
	St Giles Link Road
	Waterworld Car Park
	Wrexham General Station *(Arriva Wales)*
	'Elihu Yale', Regent Street *(JDW)*
	'Nandos', Eagles Meadow *(Nandos)*
	'North & South Wales Bank', High Street *(JDW)*
	'Yates's Bar', High Street *(Yates)*

MID & WEST WALES

Carmarthenshire

Abergorlech	Village Centre
Alltwalis	Village Centre (8.00-18.00)
Ammanford	Bus Station Car Park (9.00-18.00, later in summer)
	Carregamman Car Park (6.00-20.00)
Brechfa	Village
Burry Port	Harbour
	by Railway Station (7.30-17.00, later in summer)
Carmarthen	Carmarthen Market
	John Street Car Park (6.00-20.00)
	St Peters Car Park (6.00-20.00)
	Carmarthen Bus Station *(Private)*
	Carmarthen Station, Platform 1 *(Arriva Wales)*
	'Yr Hen Dderwen', King Street *(JDW)*
Carreg Cennen	Castle Car Park
Cenarth	Village (9.00-18.00)
Cross Hands	Bristol House, off end of M4
	Carmarthen Road, nr. Square (8.30-16.00)
Cynwyl Elfed	Village (7.30-17.30)
Ferryside	Village (7.30-19.00, later in summer)
Glanamman	Cwmamman Square (9.00-18.00, later in summer)
Gorslas	Car Park (7.30-20.00)
Kidwelly	Square (7.30-17.00, later in summer)
	Kidwelly Castle *(Cadw)*
Laugharne	below Castle (6.00-20.00)
Llanboidy	Village (8.00-17.00, later in summer))
Llanddowror	by Church (7.30-17.00)
Llandeilo	Crescent Road Car Park (6.00-20.00)
Llandovery	Castle Car Park (6.00-20.00, later in summer)
Llanelli	Island Place Bus Station (6.00-20.00)
	Provision Market (Mon-Sat 8.00-17.30)

	Parc Howard (Park hrs) Town Hall Square (6.00-20.00) North Dock Beach *(Millennium Coastal Park)* Llanelli Station *(Arriva Wales)* 'York Palace', Stepney Street *(JDW)* Pembrey Country Park Caravan Club Site *(Caravan Club)*
Llanpumsaint	Village (8.00-16.30, later in summer)
Llansaint	Welfare Hall (8.00-18.00)
Llansteffan	Car Park, South (8.00-17.30, later in summer) Green (Apr-Oct, 8.00-21.00)
Llanybydder	by Cross Hands Hotel (7.00-19.00) Car Park (5.00-18.30)
Llyn Llech Owain	Country Park (Park hrs)
Meidrim	Village Centre (7.00-17.00, later in summer)
Meinciau	Community Hall (8.00-17.30)
Newcastle Emlyn	Cattle Mart (8.30-18.00, later in summer) Cawdor Buildings
Pencader	Village (7.30-17.30)
Pendine	Car Park (7.30-18.00, later in summer) Spring Well (Apr-Oct, 7.30-22.00)
Pontwelli	by Wilkes Head (8.00-18.00)
St Clears	Car Park (6.00-22.00)
Talley	nr. Abbey
Tumble	High Street (8.30-16.00)
Velindre	Parc Puw (8.00-20.00)
Whitland	Cross Street (8.00-18.00, later in summer)

Ceredigion

Aberaeron	Masons Road North Beach Pen Cei
Aberporth	Glanmardy Penrodyn
Aberystwyth	Bath Street Castle Grounds

	Harbour
	Marine Terrace, The Shelter
	Park Avenue
	Aberystwyth Station, Platform 1 *(Arriva Wales)*
	'Varsity', Upper Portland St *(Barracuda)*
	'Yr Hen Orsaf', Alexandra Road *(JDW)*
	Glan-y-Mor Leisure Park *(Private)*
CP	Council Offices (Office hrs)
CP	Welsh Assembly Government Offices *(WA)*
Borth	by Coastguard, South Beach
	Pantyfedwyn, North Beach
	Swn-y-Mor Leisure Park *(Private)*
Cardigan/Aberteifi	Bath House
	Greenfield Car Park
	Victoria Gardens
Cenarth	Town
Devils Bridge	behind Village Shop
Lampeter	Market Street Car Park
	Rookery Lane Car Park
	St Thomas Street
Llanarth	Shawsmead Caravan Club Site *(Caravan Club)*
Llandysul	Car Park
Llangrannog	Ger y Traeth/Beachside
Llanrhystud	Pengarreg Caravan Park *(Private)*
New Quay/Cei Newydd	Paragon Car Park

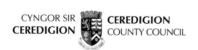

CYNGOR SIR **CEREDIGION**
CEREDIGION COUNTY COUNCIL

Contact us for a copy of our
Public Convenience Information Booklet
Glanyrafon Depot,
Glanyrafon Industrial Estate,
Aberystwyth ☎ 01970 633900
SY23 3JQ
e-mail: facilities.helpdesk@ceredigion.gov.uk

Awarded for Excellence

the disability rights people

Become a member of Radar
Network with like-minded people
and keep up to date with disability
sector news.

www.radar.org.uk

	South John Street
Penbryn	Penbryn Beach
Tregaron	Car Park
Tresaith	Ger y Traeth/Beachside

Pembrokeshire

Amroth	Amroth West
Bosherston	Car Park
Broad Haven	Marine Road
	National Park Car Park (April-October)
Burton	Jolly Sailor Car Park (April-October)
Carew	opp. The Castle
Cilgerran	Picnic Site
Cresswell Quay	Quay
Crymych	Main Road, The Square
Dale	Coronation Hall
Dinas Cross	A487 Main Road by Playing Field
Felindre Farchog	A487 Lay-by
Fishguard	The Square (Daytime)
	West Street Car Park (Daytime)
	Fishguard Ferry Terminal *(Stena)*
Freshwater	East
	West
	Freshwater East Caravan Club Site *(Caravan Club)*
Goodwick	Parrog Car Park
Gwaun Valley	[No specific information available]
Haverfordwest	Castle Lake (Daytime)
	Riverside MSCP (Daytime)
	Leisure Centre (Daytime)
	'William Owen', Quay Street *(JDW)*
Johnston	Pope Hill
Kilgetty	Tourist Information Car Park
Letterston	The Square

Little Haven	Car Park
Manorbier	Beach
Marloes	[No specific information available]
Milford Haven	Gelliswick Manchester Square (Daytime) Market Square (Daytime) The Rath (Daytime)
Moylegrove	[No specific information available]
Narberth	Towns Moor Car Park (Daytime)
Nevern	behind Old School
Newgale	Central Car Park by Duke of Edinburgh (April-October)
Newport	Long Street Car Park
Neyland	Brunel Quay Marina
Nolton Haven	[No specific information available] (Summer)
Pembroke	Commons (Daytime) Parade
Pembroke Dock	Front Street Hobbs Point (Daytime) Library (Daytime)
Penally	[No specific information available]
Penblewin	Car Park
Porthgain	[No specific information available]
St Davids	Bryn Road, behind City Hall The Grove Car Park (April-Oct, daytime) Porthclais Quickwell Hill Car Park Whitesands Beach Car Park Lleithyr Meadow Caravan Club Site *(Caravan Club)*
St Dogmaels	High Street Poppit Sands
St Florence	Village Hall *(Hall Committee)*
St Ishmaels	[No specific information available] (April-October)
St Nicholas	Village Hall, nr. Church *(Hall Committee)*

Saundersfoot	Coppit Hall Car Park (April-Oct, daytime)
	Harbour Car Park (Daytime)
	Regency Car Park (April-Oct, daytime)
Solva	Lower Car Park
Stackpole	Stackpole Quay *(National Trust)*
Stepaside	Heritage Centre (April-Oct)
Templeton	Play Area (April-October)
Tenby	Buttsfield Car Park (Daytime)
	Castle Beach (Daytime)
	MSCP (Daytime)
	North Beach
	Salterns Car Park
	South Beach (Summer, daytime)
	Upper Frog Street
Trevine	[No specific information available]
Wisemans Bridge	[No specific information available]

Powys

Abergwesyn	Community Hall (Summer) *(Community Council)*
Brecon	Lion Yard
	Produce Market (Market Days)
	Promenade, Upper Meadow
	Theatr Brycheiniog
	Brynich Caravan Club Park *(Caravan Club)*
Builth Wells	Groe Car Park
	The Strand *(Town Council)*

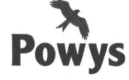

Powys

Gwasanaethau Adfywio
a'r Amgylchedd

www.powys.gov.uk
0845 607 6060

Caersws	Bridge Street
Carno	nr. Post Office
Clywedog	Y Dremfadeg, Main Dam *(Severn Trent)*
Crickhowell	Beaufort Street *(Private)*
Glasbury-on-Wye	off A438
Hay-on-Wye	Oxford Road Car Park
Knighton	Norton Arms Car Park Offa's Dyke Centre (Daytime)
Lake Vyrnwy	by Main Dam & Estate Office *(Severn Trent)*
Llananno	A483, between Crossgates & Newtown
Llanbrynmair	Car Park
Llandrindod Wells	Lakeside (Daytime) Station Crescent Town Hall Grounds 'The Metropole', Temple Street *(Private)*
Llanfair Caereinion	Bridge Street
Llanfihangell-yng-Ngwynfa	Car Park *(Community Council)*
Llanfyllin	High Street, opp. Car Park
Llangorse Common	Car Park
Llangynog	Car Park
Llanidloes	Gro Car Park
Llanrhaeadr-ym-Mochnant	Village Waterfall
Llansantffraed	A40, west of Bwlch
Llansanffraidd	A495 Main Road
Llanspyddid	A40, west of Brecon
Llanwrtyd Wells	nr. New Inn
Machynlleth	Maengwyn Street Car Park Machynlleth Station *(Arriva Wales)*
Meifod	Car Park
Newtown	Back Lane Car Park Gravel Car Park
Pen-y-Cae	Craig-y-Nos Country Pk *(Brecon Beacons NP)*

Presteigne	Hereford Street
	Wilson Terrace (Daytime) *(Town Council)*
Rhayader	Dark Lane
Sennybridge	High Street
Storey Arms	A470, between Brecon & Merthyr
Talgarth	The Square
Welshpool	Berriew Street Car Park
	Church Street Car Park
Ystradfellte	Porth-yr-Ogof Car Park *(Brecon Beacons NP)*
Ystrydgynlais	The Cross

SOUTH WALES

Blaenau Gwent

Abertillery	Tillery Street
	'Pontlottyn', Somerset Street *(JDW)*
Blaina	Blaina Cemetery (Daytime)
	Cwmcelyn Road
Cwm	Cwm Cemetery (Daytime)
Brynmawr	Brynmawr Cemetery (Daytime)
	Market Square
Ebbw Vale	Ebbw Vale Cemetery (Daytime)
	Market Street
	'Picture House', Market Street *(JDW)*
Tredegar	Cefn Golau Cemetery (Daytime)
	Dukestown Cemetery (Daytime)
	Gwent Shopping Centre *(Private)*
	'Olympia', Morgan Street *(JDW)*

Bridgend

Bridgend	Brackla Street, Cheapside
	Bridgend Bus Station
	Derwen Road (9.00-18.00)
	Bridgend Station, Platform 1 *(Arriva Wales)*
	'Dunraven Arms', Derwen Road *(Private)*
	'Ikon Nightclub', Nolton Street *(Private)*

For more information on public
facilities and access at many
attractions, why not telephone
before you travel?

Please telephone for all enquiries:

01495 311 556

For more information on Toilet
Facilities and access at all Local
Attractions, why not telephone for
details before you travel?
Please telephone for all enquiries:

01656 643443

'Lava Lounge', Nolton Street *(Private)*
'Litten Tree', opp. Bus Station *(Private)*
'O'Neils', Nolton Street *(Private)*
'Tuskers Bar', Wyndham Street *(Private)*
'West House', Cefn Glas *(Private)*
'Wyndham Arms', Dunraven Place *(JDW)*

Maesteg	Maesteg Bus Station
Porthcawl	Griffin Park
	John Street
	Rest Bay Car Park
	High Tide Inn, Mackworth Road
Ton Kenfig	Kenfig Nature Reserve (9.00-17.00)

Caerphilly

Bargoed	Bus Terminus, Hanbury Square [to be redeveloped]
Blackwood	Bus Station (Daytime, Mon-Sat)
	'The Sirhowy', High Street *(JDW)*
Caerphilly	Bus/Railway Terminus (8.00-19.30)
	Lower Twyn, Tourist Inf. Office (8.00-19.30)
Crosskeys	Sirhowy Valley Country Park
Deri	Parc Cwm Darren (2) (April-Oct)
Nelson	Bus Station
Newbridge	High Street
Oakdale	Pen Y Fan Pond Country Park (April-Oct)
Risca	Tredegar Street
Ystrad Mynach	Bedlwyn Road, by Bus Terminus

Cardiff

Canton	Delta Street
	Pontcanna Caravan Site (Site users)
	Sophia Gardens Car Park (9.00-16.00)
Cardiff City Centre	Frederick Street
	The Hayes
	Britannia Park (Daytime) *(Port Authority)*
	Havannah Street (Daytime) *(Port Authority)*
	Capitol Shopping Centre *(Private)*

Queens Arcade Shopping Centre *(Private)*
St Davids Shopping Centre *(Private)*
CP St Davids 2 Shopping Centre *(Private)*
Debenhams Store, St Davids Way *(Debenhams)*
Cardiff Central Station, Subway *(Arriva Wales)*
Queen Street Station, Platform 1 *(Arriva Wales)*
'Cayo Arms', Cathedral Road *(Private)*
'Crockerton', Greyfriars Road *(JDW)*
'Dewi's', Mary Ann Street *(Private)*
'Edwards', St Marys Street *(M&B)*
'Gatekeeper', Westgate Street *(JDW)*
'Great Western', St Mary Street *(JDW)*
'Ha! Ha! Bar', Greyfriars Road *(Private)*
'The Halfway', Cathedral Road *(Private)*
'Ivor Davis', Cowbridge Road East *(JDW)*
'Jongleurs', Millennium Plaza *(Private)*
'Moloko', Mill Lane *(Private)*
'Nandos', Bute Street, Mermaid Quay *(Nandos)*
'Nandos', St Davids Centre *(Nandos)*
'Nandos', St Marys Street *(Nandos)*
'Old Orleans', Church Street *(Private)*

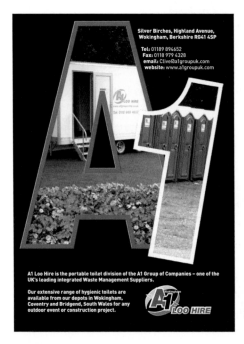
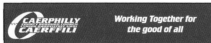

'O'Neills', St Marys Street *(M&B)*
'Philharmonic', St Marys Street *(Prvate)*
'Prince of Wales', St Mary Street *(JDW)*
'Que Pasa', Trinity St *(Marstons)*
'Robins Bar', Cowbridge Road East *(Private)*
'Varsity', Greyfriars Road *(Barracuda)*
'Walkabout', St Marys Street *(Private)*
Millennium Stadium (Match & Event Days) *(Private)*
St David's Hall (Hall hrs) *(Private)*
SWALEC Stadium *(Glamorgan Cricket)*
CP National Assembly Building (Building hrs) *(WA)*

Cathays	Whitchurch Road, by Library (Park hrs)
	CP National Museum of Wales, Cathays Park (Museum hrs)
Lisvane	Cefn-on-Park, Cherry Orchard Rd (Park hrs)
Llandaff	Llandaff Fields, Cathedral Road
Llanishen	Ty Glas Road
Plasnewydd	Albany Road
	Roath Park, Boatstage (Park hrs)
	Roath Park, Rose Gardens (Park hrs)
	'Central Bar', Windsor Place *(JDW)*
	'Ernest Willows', City Road *(JDW)*
	'Varsity', *199 Richmond Road (Barracuda)*
Rhiwbina	Heol y Deri
St Fagans	**CP** National History Museum (Museum hrs)
Thompson Park	Romilly Road (Park hrs)

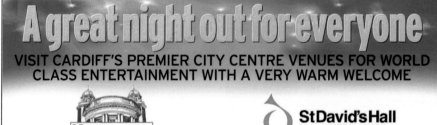
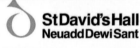

Victoria Park	Cowbridge Road East (Park hrs)
	Victoria Park, Paddling Pool (Park hrs)
	Western Cemetery (Cemetery hrs)
Whitchurch	Penlline Road

Merthyr Tydfil

Dowlais		Dowlais Shopping Centre (M+F) (9.00-17.00)
Llwyn-On	CP	Garwnant Visitor Centre (Centre hrs)
Merthyr Tydfil		Bus Station (9.00-18.00)
		Cyfarthfa Park (Park hrs)
		by Shopmobility, behind Police Station
		St Tydfils Square (9.00-18.00) *(Private)*
		'Nandos', Rhydycar Leisure Complex *(Nandos)*
		'Y Dic Penderyn', High Street *(JDW)*

Monmouthshire

Abergavenny	Castle Street Car Park
	Market Hall (Market hrs)
	Old Bus Station Car Park
	Whitehorse Lane
	'Coliseum', Lion Street *(JDW)*
	Pandy Caravan Club Site *(Caravan Club)*
Caldicot	Caldicot Castle Country Park
Chepstow	Bank Street
	Bridge Street Car Park
	Bulwark, by Severn Bridge Social Club
	Riverside
Gilwern	Abergavenny Road
Grosmont	Village Square
Llanthony	Llanthony Abbey Picnic Site
	Llanthony Priory Car Park *(Brecon Beacons NP)*
Mitchell Troy	Picnic Site, A449 Northbound
Monmouth	Cattle Market
	Waitrose Supermarket, Monnow Street *(Private)*
	'King's Head', Agincourt Square *(JDW)*
Raglan	Castle Street
Tintern	Beaufort Cottage, The Abbey

Usk	Maryport Street Car Park
	The Island Usk Picnic Site, A472

Neath Port Talbot

Aberdulais	Aberdulais Falls *(National Trust)*
Briton Ferry	by Library, Neath Road
	Lodge Court
Dyffryn Cellwen	Main Road
Neath	Banwen Road, Glyneath
	Market
	Victoria Gardens
	Neath Station, Platform 1 *(Arriva Wales)*
	'David Protheroe', Windsor Road *(JDW)*
Pontardawe	Herbert Street Car Park
Port Talbot	Bus Station
	Princess Margaret Way, Sandfields
	Western Avenue, Sandfields
	Port Talbot Parkway Station *(Arriva Wales)*
	'Lord Caradoc', Station Road *(JDW)*
Resolven	Canal Car Park
Skewen	Queens Road

Newport

Bettws	Bettws Shopping Centre
Caerleon	Cricket Pavilion, The Broadway (Daytime)
	High Street (Daytime)
Maindee	Chepstow Road, opp Police Station (Daytime)
Newport	Caerleon Road, by The Victoria (Daytime)
	Cardiff Road, opp Police Station
	Corporation Road, entrance to park (Daytime)
	Newport Provision Market (Market hrs)
	Kingsway Shopping Centre *(Private)*
	Newport Station *(Arriva Wales)*
	'Godfrey Morgan', Chepstow Road *(JDW)*
	'Tom Toya Lewis', Commercial Street *(JDW)*
	'John Wallace Linton', Cambrian Centre *(JDW)*
	Tredegar House Caravan Club Site *(Caravan Club)*

Rhondda Cynon Taf

Aberaman	Cardiff Road
Aberdare	Bus Station, Duke Street Monk Street 'Yr Iuean Ap Iago', High Street *(JDW)*
Cwmaman	Alexandra Terrace. Fforchaman Road
Maerdy	Maerdy Park
Mountain Ash	Oxford Street
Nantgarw	'Nandos', Treforest Ind. Estate *(Nandos)* Nantgarw BowlPlex, Treforest Ind. Estate *(BowlPlex)*
Pentre	Bridgend Square
Pontyclun M4	Cardiff West Services, J33 M4 *(Moto)*
Pontypridd	Bus Station, Morgan Street Sardis Road Pontypridd Station, Platform 1 *(Arriva Wales)* 'Tumble Inn', Broadway *(JDW)*
Porth	Hannah Street
Talbot Green	Bus Depot, Talbot Road
Tonypandy	Dunraven Street
Treherbert	Bute Street
Treorchy	nr. Parc & Dare Theatre, Station Road
Ynysybwl	Windsor Place

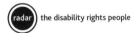
the disability rights people

Visit Radar's online shop

For a range of products to promote independent living.

www.radar-shop.org.uk

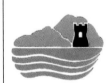

Neath Port Talbot County Borough Council Directorate of Environment

Neath Port Talbot County Borough Council is committed to supporting the RADAR key programme for access to all its toilets with Disabled Facilities

Swansea

Blackpill	Blackpill Lido, off Mumbles Road
Bracelet Bay	Car Park
Caswell Bay	off Caswell Road, Car Park
Gorseinon	West Street, by Bus Station
Gowerton	Gowerton Caravan Club Site *(Caravan Club)*
Horton	Car Park
Llansamlet	'Dylan Thomas', Samlet Road *(Private)*
Morriston	Woodfield Street, nr, Church
Mumbles	Oystermouth Square
Penllegaer M4	Swansea Services, M4 Junct 47 *(Moto)*
Pontardulais	Water Street
Port Eynon	Foreshore Car Park
Rhossili	nr. Hotel
Swansea	Caer Street, off Princess Way

CP Civic Centre, Oystermouth Road (Office hrs)
Guildhall, Guildhall Road South (Office hrs)
Liberty Stadium (Match Days)
Marina, Maritime Quarter
Marina, Trawler Road
Quadrant Bus Station
Welcome Lane, off Castle Street
Quandrant Shopping Centre, 1st Floor *(Private)*
Debenhams Store, The Quadrant *(Debenhams)*
Swansea Station, Platform 4 *(Arriva Wales)*
'Bank Statement', Wind Street *(JDW)*
'Nandos', Wind Street *(Nandos)*
'Potters Wheel', Kingsway *(JDW)*
'Square', Wind Street *(Private)*
'Varsity', Wind Street/Castle Square *(Barracuda)*
'Walkabout', Castle Square *(Private)*
'Yates's Bar', Caer Street *(Yates)*
CP LC Leisure Centre, Oystermouth Rd *(Private)*

Torfaen

Cwmbran	Cwmbran Station *(Arriva Wales)*
	'John Fielding', Caradoc Road *(JDW)*
	Cwmbran BowlPlex, Glyndwr Rd *(BowlPlex)*
Pontypool	Indoor Market (Market hrs)
	'John Capel Hanbury', Osborne Rd *(JDW)*

Vale Of Glamorgan

Barry	Court Road/Holton Road MSCP
	Knap Car Terrace, Bron y Mor
	Park Crescent, Romilly Road
	Porthkerry Country Park, Café Car Park
	Thomson Street, by Home Bargains
	Tynewydd Road, by Library (Daytime)
	Weston Square, Vere St/Gladstone Rd
	Netto Store, Thomson Street *(Netto)*
	'Sir Samuel Romilly', Romilly Building *(JDW)*
Barry Island	Barry Island Car Park, Clive Road
	Western Shelter, Paget Road
Cowbridge	**CP** Cowbridge Leisure Centre (Centre hrs)
	Town Hall Car Park, High Street
Llantwit Major	Boverton Rd, Pound Field Shopping Centre
	Cwm Colhuw, Llantwit Major Beach
	Town Hall Car Park, The Square
Ogmore by Sea	Car Park, off Main Road
Penarth	Albert Road/West Terrace
	Cosmeston Village, Lavernock Road
	The Esplanade, Italian Gardens
	The Esplanade, Penarth Pier
	CP Penarth Leisure Centre (Centre hrs)
	'Bears Head', Windsor Road *(JDW)*
Southerndown	Dunraven Beach opp. Car Park

Antrim

Antrim	Castle Centre Car Park (M+F)
	Antrim Bus Station *(Translink)*
	Antrim Station *(Translink)*
	Antrim Campus *(Northern Regional College))*
Crumlin Glen	Car Park, by bridge

Ards

Ballyhalbert	Harbour Road, Car Park
Ballywalter	Springvale Road, by Tennis Courts
Comber	Castle Street Car Park
	Islandhill Car Park, Ringhaddy Road
Cloughey	Warren Car Park, Main Road
Donaghadee	The Commons Pavilion, Millisle Road
	The Parade (8.00-18.00, later in summer)
Greyabbey	Main Street
Killinchy	Whiterock Picnic Area, Ballydorn Road
Millisle	Ballywalter Road Car Park
Newtownards	Mill Street
	Newtownards Bus Station *(Translink)*
	'Spirit Merchant', Regent Street *(JDW)*

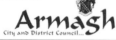
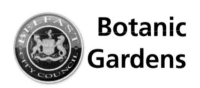

Botanic Gardens

Open all year round

Free Admission

| Portaferry | Castle Park, by Exploris |
| Portavogie | Anchor Car Park, Springvale Road |

Armagh

Armagh	Armagh Bus Station *(Translink)*
	CP Armagh Leisure Centre (Centre hrs)
Markethill	The Square
Tandragee	Market Street

Ballymena

Ballymena	Ballymena Bus/Rail Station *(Translink)*
	CAFÉ Lamont *(Northern Regional College)*
	Farm Lodge Buildings *(Northern Regional College)*
	Trostan Ave. Buildings *(Northern Regional College)*
	'Spinning Mill', Broughshane Street *(JDW)*

Banbridge

Banbridge	Corbet Lough, Aughnacloy Road
	Kenlis Street
	New Cemetery, Newry Road
	CP Southern Regional College (College hrs)
Dromore	Dromore Park, Banbridge Road
	Market Square
Katesbridge	Katesbridge Picnic Area
Loughbrickland	Village Park, Poynzpass Road
Scarva	Main Street
	Old Mill Road, Scarva Park

Belfast

Central Belfast	Arthur Lane, Arthur Street (Daytime)
	Bankmore Square, Dublin Road
	Botanic Gardens (Park hrs)
	Church Lane, Ann Street (Daytime)
	Custom House Square
	Lombard Street
	St Georges Market (Market hours)
	Winetavern Street (Daytime)
	Europa Buscentre *(Translink)*

Laganside Buscentre *(Translink)*
Belfast Botanic Station *(Translink)*
Central Station *(Translink)*
Great Victoria Street Station *(Translink)*
Debenhams Store, Castle Court *(Debenhams)*
'Bridge House', Bedford Street *(JDW)*
'Nandos', Bedford Street *(Nandos)*
'Nandos', Victoria Street *(Nandos)*

East Belfast

Connswater, Westminster Ave (Mon-Sat, Daytime)
CP George Best Belfast City Airport *(Private)*

North Belfast

Agnes Street (Mon-Sat, Daytime)
Waterworks, Antrim Road
Yorkgate Station *(Translink)*

South Belfast

Cranmore Park, Lisburn Road (Park Hrs)
Drumglass Park, Lisburn Road (Daytime)
Gasworks, Ormeau Road
Ormeau Embankment, Ormeau Bridge (Daytime)
Roselawn Cemetery (Cemetery hrs)
Sir Thomas & Lady Dixon Park (Park hrs)
Stormont Estate (Park hrs)

West Belfast

CP Divis & Black Mountain Centre *(National Trust)*

Carrickfergus

Carrickfergus

Harbour Car Park, by Castle
Carrickfergus Station *(Translink)*
'Central Bar', High Street *(JDW)*

Whitehead

Whitehead Car Park
Whitehead Station *(Translink)*

Coleraine

Castlerock

Promenade (May-Sept)
Hezlett House *(National Trust)*

Coleraine

Long Commons
Park Street
Railway Road, Leisure Centre Car Park
Strand Road, Riverside Park
Coleraine Bus/Rail Station *(Translink)*
'Old Court House', Castlerock Road *(JDW)*

Downhill	Downhill Beach Car Park (May-Sept)
Garvagh	Bridge Street
Kilrea	Garvagh Road
Portballintrae	Beach Road Car Park The Harbour (May-Sept)
Portrush	Arcadia (May-Sept) Dunluce Avenue Strand Road, Riverside Park Whiterocks Car Park (May-Sept)
Portstewart	Harbour Road

Cookstown

Cookstown	Burn Road Bus Station *(Translink)*

Craigavon

Lurgan	Castle Lane
Portadown	William Street *(Portadown 2000)* Portadown Station *(Translink)*

Carrickfergus Borough

Town Hall
Carrickfergus
Co Antrim BT38 7DL

Tel: 02893 358000
Fax: 02893 366676

SUPPORTING THE WORK
OF RADAR AND THE
NATIONAL KEY SCHEME

COLERAINE

COLERAINE BOROUGH COUNCIL

For more information on access to our public facilities
and advice on where to purchase a RADAR key please
contact us using the details below:

Coleraine Borough Council
Cloonavin
66 Portstewart Road
Coleraine
Co. Londonderry
BT52 1EY

Web: www.colerainebc.gov.uk
Email: technical@colerainebc.gov.uk

Derry

Derry	Victoria Car Park, Strand Road
	Bus Station, Foyle Street *(Translink)*
	Waterside Railway Station *(Translink)*
	Debenhams Store, Foyleside *(Debenhams)*
	Sainsbury's Store, Strand Road *(Sainsbury)*
	'The Diamond', Diamond *(JDW)*
	'Ice Wharf', Strand Road *(JDW)*

Down

Ardglass	The Harbour
Ballyhornan	Rocks Road
Castlewellan	Upper Square
Crossgar	Killyleagh Street
Downpatrick	Market Street
	Downpatrick Bus Station *(Translink)*
Dundrum	Picnic Area, Newcastle Road
Killyleagh	Delamont Country Park (Park hrs)
	High Street

Craigavon Borough Council

For more information on
Public Facilities and Access
at many attractions, why not
telephone for more details
before you travel?

Please telephone for all
enquiries: 02838 312400

DERRY CITY COUNCIL

Council Offices
98 Strand Road
Derry BT48 7NN

Telephone 028 7136 3569
Fax 028 7136 3569

DERRY CITY COUNCIL SUPPORT
THE PROVISION OF FACILITIES
FOR ALL ITS CITIZENS

Newcastle	Central Promenade
	Donard Park
	Downs Road
	Islands Park
	South Promenade
	Bus Station *(Translink)*
Quoile	Car Park
Saintfield	New Line

Dungannon & South Tyrone

Augher	Clogher Road
Ballygawley	Church Street
Coalisland	Lineside
Dungannon	Scotch Street
	Dungannon Bus Station *(Translink)*
Fivemiletown	Main Street
Moy	Charlemont Street
Peatlands Park	Visitor Centre *(Natural Heritage)*

Fermanagh

| Enniskillen | Enniskillen Bus Station *(Translink)* |
| | 'Linen Hall', Townhall Street *(JDW)* |

Larne

| Larne | Larne Bus Station *(Translink)* |
| | Larne Station *(Translink)* |

Limavady

Benone	Beach (Seasonal)
Dungiven	Main Street
Limavady	Catherine Street
	Main Street
	Bus Station *(Translink)*
Roe Valley Country Park	Dogleap Centre *(Natural Heritage)*

Lisburn

Hillsborough		Ballynahinch Street
Lisburn	**CP**	Civic Centre, Lagan Valley Island
		Lisburn Bus Station *(Translink)*
		Lisburn Station *(Translink)*
		'Tuesday Bell'. Lisburn Square *(JDW)*

Magherafelt

Draperstown	Derrynoid Road
Magherafelt	Magherafelt Bus Station *(Translink)*
	Magherafelt Campus *(Northern Regional College)*

Moyle

Armoy	Main Street
Ballintoy	Harbour
Ballycastle	Harbour Car Park
	Quay Road Pavilion
	Seafront Centre
Bushmills	Dundrave

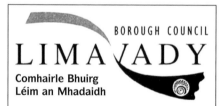

BOROUGH COUNCIL

LIMA√ADY

Comhairle Bhuirg
Léim an Mhadaidh

Limavady Borough Council
provides access for and awareness
of people with disabilties throughout
all its premises, and incorporates
the National RADAR Key Scheme
in various public conveniences
throughout the Borough

For further information please contact:
Limavardy Borough Council
7 Connell Street, Limavady
Northern Ireland BT49 0HA
T. 028 777 60305   F. 028 777 29005
www.limavady.gov.uk

For information on obtaining
RADAR keys for public
convenience facilities please
contact customer services on:

(028) 30313233

Newry & Mourne District Council
Haughey House, Rampart Road
Greenback Industrial Estate,
Newry, BT34 2QU
Tel: (028) 3031 3233 Fax: (028) 3031 3299
Minicom: (028) 3025 7859
www.newryandmourne.gov.uk
Email: techleisure@newryandmourne.gov.uk

	Giants Causeway Visitor Centre
Cushendall	Legg Green
	Mill Street Car Park
	Waterford Slipway
Cushendun	Beach Car Park
Dunservick	Harbour
Rathlin Island	Church Bay
Waterfoot	Main Street

Newry & Mourne

Annalong	Marine Park (Daytime)
Bloodybridge	Amenity Area (Daytime)
Crossmaglen	Loughross Amenity Area (M+F) (Daytime)
	The Square (Daytime)
Hilltown	Rostrevor Road (Daytime)
	Spelga Amenity Area (M+F) (Apr-Oct, daytime)
Kilkeel	Lower Square (Daytime)
	Cranfield Beach (M+F) (April-Oct, daytime)

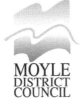

MOYLE DISTRICT COUNCIL

We are delighted to say that all our disabled toilets within the **Moyle District Council** area are fitted with the **RADAR** lock and we are proud to be a member of the association.

Best wishes to Radar from
Door-2-Door Transport
Northern Ireland
Tel: 0845 9 800 800

	Greencastle Street (M+F) (Daytime)
Newry	Newry Market, Hill Street (8.00-18.00)
	Newry Sports Centre, Patrick's St (Centre hrs)
	Newry Town Hall, Bank Parade
	Bus Station *(Translink)*
	Newry Station *(Translink)*
Rostrevor	The Square (M+F) (8.00-18.00)
Warrenpoint	The Park, Queen Street (M+F) (Daytime)
	The Square (M+F) (Daytime)

Newtownabbey

Ballyclare	Main Street (7.30-dusk)
	Sixmilewater River Park (8.00-dusk)
	Ballyclare Bus Station *(Translink)*
Jordanstown	Loughshore Park, Shore Road (8.00-dusk)
Newtownabbey	Newtownabbey Bus Station *(Translink)*
Whiteabbey	Hazelbank Park, Shore Road (8.00-dusk)

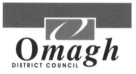

Omagh
DISTRICT COUNCIL

Council Offices, The Grange
Mountjoy Road, Omagh
Co Tyrone BT79 7BL

Tel: 02882 245 321
Fax: 02882 243 888

**Supporting the work of RADAR
and the National Key Scheme**

Strabane
District Council
Comhairle Ceantair
an tSratha Báin
Stràbane Destrick Cooneil

The following public conveniences fitted with **Radar** locks can be found in the list below:

Castlederg, William Street
Cranagh, Glenelly Road
Newtownstewart, Main Street
Plumbridge, Fair Green
Strabane, Market Street
Sion Mills, Melmount Road

Strabane District Council, 47 Derry Road
Strabane, Co. Tyrone, N. Ireland BT82 8DY
Tel: 028 7138 2204 Fax: 028 7138 1343

Email: admin@strabanedc.com
Website: www.strabanedc.com

North Down

Bangor	Abbey Street Car Park, opp. Bus Station
	Ballyholme Park, Ballyholme Esplanade
	Banks Lane Car Park, Groomsport Road
	McKee Clock, Quay Street
	Pickie Fun Park, Marine Gardens
	Ward Park, Park Drive
	Bangor Bus/Rail Station *(Translink)*
	Crawfordsburn Country Park
	Beach Car Park *(Natural Heritage)*
	Helens Bay Car Park *(Natural Heritage)*
Groomsport	Harbour Road
Holywood	Hibernia Street
	Seapark Recreation Area

Omagh

Beragh	Main Street
Dromore	Alexander Terrace
Omagh	Johnston Park/Kevlin Avenue
	Scarff's Entry (Daytime)
	Omagh Bus Station (Translink)
Sixmilecross	Main Street
Trillick	Main Street

Strabane

Castlederg	William Street
Cranagh	Glenelly Road
Donemana	Berryhill Road
Newtownstewart	Main Street
Plumbridge	Fair Green
Sion Mills	Melmount Road
Strabane	Market Street
	Strabane Bus Station *(Translink)*

CHANNEL ISLANDS

Guernsey

Castel	Grande Rocque Beach
	Saumarez Park
	Vazon Beach
St Martins	Icart
	Jerbourg Car Park
	Moulin Huet Bay Car Park
St Peter Port	Bus Terminus
	Castle Emplacement
	Crown Pier
	Market Square
	North Beach Car Park
	St Julians Avenue
	White Rock Ferry Terminal
St Peters	L'Erée Beach

St Sampson's	Delancy Park South Side
Vale	Bordeaux Beach
	Chouet Beach
	North Side, The Bridge

Jersey

Grouville	Gorey Common
	La Rocque (M+F)
St Brelades	Corbiere
	La Pulante
	Le Haule
	Ouaisne
	Red Houses
	St Aubins
	Underground, St Brelades Bay
	Woodford, St Brelades Bay
St Clements	La Mare (M+F)
	Le Hocq
	Millards Corner (M+F)

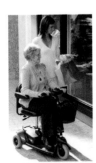

St Helier	First Tower
	Liberation Bus Station
	Minden Place, Car Park
	Patriotic Street, Car Park
	Sand Street Car Park
	Snow Hill Car Park (M+F) {under review}
St John	Bonne Nuit
St Lawrence	Bel Royal
	Millbrook, Promenade
	Millbrook, Coromation Park (Park hrs)
St Martin	Archirondel
	Gorey House
	St Catherines
St Ouens	Greve De Lecq
	Le Braye
	Les Laveurs
St Peters	Beaumont, Gunsite
Trinity	Rozel

Douglas	Drumgold Street Car Park
	Jubilee Clock, Loch Promenade
	Loch Promenade Gardens
	Nobles Park, St Ninian Road
	Shaw Brow Car Park, Barrack St
	York Road
	'Colours', Central Promenade *(Private)*
	'Fiesta Havana', Wellington Street *(Private)*
Laxey	The Harbour
Onchan	Port Jack
	Onchan Pleasure Park *(Private)*
Peel	Market Place
	Shore Road/Victoria Road
	Peel Camp Site *(Private)*
Ramsey	Bowring Road
	Coronation Park
	Market Place
	Mooragh Park, Lakeside Pavilion
	Ramsey Town Library (Library hrs)
St Johns	Main Road

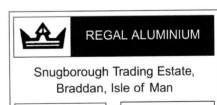

INDEX OF ADVERTISERS

Radar thanks all its advertisers for supporting the publication of its books for disabled people.

INDEX OF LOCALITIES

A

B

INDEX OF LOCALITIES

C

D

E

H

M

N

O

P

S

T

U

V

W

Y